*Welcome to the **"5 Ingredient Cookbook for Men: Cooking Hacks for Men Who Hate Complicated Recipes"**! This book is designed for those who appreciate great food but don't have hours to spend in the kitchen. Whether you're a complete novice or a seasoned home cook looking to simplify your culinary adventures, this cookbook is your ticket to delicious, no-fuss meals.*

We get it. Life is busy, and spending hours slaving over a stove isn't everyone's idea of fun. That's why we've curated a collection of recipes that require just five key ingredients, without sacrificing flavor or satisfaction. From hearty dinners to impressive desserts, each recipe in this book has been carefully crafted to deliver maximum taste with minimal effort.

Inside these pages, you'll find straightforward instructions, handy cooking tips, and practical advice aimed specifically at men who want to eat well without the hassle of complicated recipes. Whether you're cooking for yourself, impressing a date, or hosting a gathering with friends, our goal is to make your time in the kitchen enjoyable and rewarding.

*So, grab your apron and let's get cooking! With the **"5 Ingredient Cookbook for Men"** in hand, you'll soon discover how easy and enjoyable cooking can be. Whether you're grilling, baking, or sautéing your way through these pages, you'll find that simplicity and flavor go hand in hand. Cheers to good food, good times, and mastering the art of cooking with ease.*

1. Avocado Toast:
Whole grain bread, avocado, lemon juice, salt, pepper.

Ingredient:

- 2 slices whole grain bread
- 1 ripe avocado, mashed
- 1 tbsp fresh lemon juice
- Salt and pepper to taste

Instructions:

1. Toast the whole grain bread until lightly golden brown.

2. In a small bowl, mash the avocado with the lemon juice. Season with salt and pepper to taste.

3. Spread the mashed avocado evenly over the toasted bread slices.

4. Serve immediately and enjoy!

You can customize this recipe by adding other toppings like sliced tomatoes, crumbled feta, red pepper flakes, or a drizzle of olive oil. The key is the creamy avocado paired with the crunchy toast and bright lemon flavor.

2. Greek Yogurt Parfait:
Greek yogurt, honey, granola, berries, chia seeds.

Ingredient:

- 1 cup plain Greek yogurt
- 2 tbsp honey
- 1/2 cup granola
- 1 cup mixed berries (such as blueberries, raspberries, strawberries)
- 1 tbsp chia seeds

Instructions:

1. In a parfait glass or bowl, layer the ingredients in the following order:

  - 1/4 cup Greek yogurt
  - 1 tbsp honey
  - 2 tbsp granola
  - 1/4 cup mixed berries
  - 1/2 tbsp chia seeds

2. Repeat the layers until you reach the top of the glass/bowl.

3. Serve chilled and enjoy!

The Greek yogurt provides protein, the honey adds sweetness, the granola gives a crunchy texture, the berries add antioxidants and fiber, and the chia seeds are a source of omega•3s. This parfait makes for a healthy, delicious, and satisfying breakfast or snack.

3. Spinach and Feta Omelette:
Eggs, spinach, feta cheese, salt, pepper.

Ingredient:

- 3 eggs
- 1 cup fresh spinach, chopped
- 1/4 cup crumbled feta cheese
- Salt and pepper to taste

Instructions:

1. Crack the eggs into a bowl and beat them lightly with a fork or whisk until well combined.

2. Heat a non•stick skillet over medium heat and spray with cooking spray.

3. Pour the beaten eggs into the skillet and let them sit for 30 seconds to a minute, until the bottom starts to set.

4. Sprinkle the chopped spinach and crumbled feta cheese over the top of the eggs.

5. Use a spatula to gently fold the omelette in half, then slide it onto a plate.

6. Season with salt and pepper to taste.

Enjoy your fresh and flavorful Spinach and Feta Omelette!

4. Banana Oat Pancakes:
Bananas, oats, eggs, baking powder, cinnamon.

Ingredient:

- 1 ripe banana, mashed
- 1 cup rolled oats
- 2 eggs
- 1 tsp baking powder
- 1/2 tsp ground cinnamon
- Pinch of salt (optional)

Instructions:

1. In a medium bowl, mash the banana until smooth.

2. Add the rolled oats, eggs, baking powder, cinnamon, and salt (if using). Stir until well combined.

3. Heat a lightly oiled skillet or griddle over medium heat.

4. Scoop about 1/4 cup of the batter onto the hot surface and cook for 2•3 minutes per side, or until golden brown.

5. Serve the banana oat pancakes warm, with your favorite toppings such as maple syrup, fresh fruit, or a dollop of yogurt.

Enjoy your homemade banana oat pancakes!

5. Berry Smoothie:
Mixed berries, Greek yogurt, honey, almond milk, ice.

Ingredient:

- 1 cup mixed berries (such as strawberries, blueberries, raspberries)
- 1/2 cup Greek yogurt
- 1•2 tbsp honey (to taste)
- 1/2 cup unsweetened almond milk
- 1 cup ice cubes

Instructions:

1. Add all the ingredients to a blender.

2. Blend on high speed until smooth and creamy.

3. Taste and adjust sweetness with more honey if desired.

4. Pour into a glass and enjoy!

This smoothie is a great way to pack in nutrients from the mixed berries, protein from the Greek yogurt, and creaminess from the almond milk. The honey adds a touch of sweetness. Feel free to adjust the amounts of each ingredient to suit your taste preferences.

6. Peanut Butter Banana Toast: Whole grain bread, peanut butter, banana, chia seeds, honey.

Ingredient:

- 2 slices whole grain bread
- 2 tablespoons peanut butter
- 1 ripe banana, sliced
- 1 teaspoon chia seeds
- 1 teaspoon honey (optional)

Instructions:

1. Toast the whole grain bread until lightly golden brown.

2. Spread the peanut butter evenly over the toasted bread.

3. Arrange the sliced banana on top of the peanut butter.

4. Sprinkle the chia seeds over the banana slices.

5. Drizzle the honey over the top, if desired.

This makes a nutritious and delicious breakfast or snack. The peanut butter provides protein, the banana adds natural sweetness and potassium, the chia seeds are a source of fiber and omega•3s, and the honey adds a touch of sweetness. Enjoy!

7. Scrambled Eggs with Salsa:
Eggs, salsa, salt, pepper, olive oil.

Ingredient:

- 6 eggs
- 2 tbsp milk or water
- 1/4 tsp salt
- 1/4 tsp black pepper
- 1 tbsp butter or oil
- 1/2 cup salsa (your favorite variety)

Instructions:

1. Crack the eggs into a medium bowl. Add the milk or water, salt, and pepper. Whisk the eggs until well blended.

2. Heat a nonstick skillet over medium heat and melt the butter or heat the oil.

3. Pour the egg mixture into the hot skillet. As the eggs begin to set around the edges, use a spatula to gently push the cooked eggs towards the center, tilting the pan to allow the uncooked egg to flow to the edges.

4. Continue cooking, stirring and folding the eggs gently, until they are softly scrambled and no longer runny, about 2•3 minutes total.

5. Remove the skillet from the heat and stir in the salsa. Serve the scrambled eggs with salsa immediately.

Enjoy your flavorful scrambled eggs with a kick of salsa! The salsa adds a nice pop of flavor and moisture to the eggs.

8. Overnight Oats:
Rolled oats, almond milk, chia seeds, honey, berries.

Ingredient:

- 1 cup rolled oats
- 1 cup unsweetened almond milk
- 1 tbsp chia seeds
- 1 tbsp honey (or maple syrup)
- 1/2 cup mixed berries (such as blueberries, raspberries, strawberries)

Instructions:

1. In a medium bowl or mason jar, combine the rolled oats, almond milk, chia seeds, and honey. Stir well to combine.

2. Cover the bowl or seal the mason jar and refrigerate overnight, or for at least 6 hours.

3. In the morning, give the overnight oats a good stir. Top with the mixed berries.

4. Enjoy the chilled, creamy overnight oats straight from the fridge. The oats will have absorbed the almond milk and become soft and puddlng•like.

Optional Variations:

- Use different types of milk (dairy, soy, coconut, etc.)
- Add a sprinkle of cinnamon or nutmeg
- Top with chopped nuts, shredded coconut, or a drizzle of peanut butter

The chia seeds provide extra fiber and nutrients, while the honey adds a touch of sweetness. The berries provide a refreshing, fruity element. This make•ahead breakfast is perfect for busy mornings!

9. Apple Cinnamon Oatmeal:
Oats, apple, cinnamon, honey, almond milk.

Ingredient:

- 1 cup rolled oats
- 1 cup unsweetened almond milk
- 1 medium apple, peeled, cored and diced
- 1 tsp ground cinnamon
- 1 tbsp honey (or maple syrup)
- Pinch of salt

Instructions:

1. In a medium saucepan, combine the rolled oats and almond milk. Bring to a simmer over medium heat, stirring occasionally.

2. Once the oats have started to thicken, about 5 minutes, stir in the diced apple, cinnamon, honey, and a pinch of salt.

3. Continue cooking, stirring frequently, until the oats are creamy and the apple is tender, about 5•7 minutes more.

4. Remove from heat and serve the apple cinnamon oatmeal warm.

5. You can top it with additional honey, a splash of almond milk, chopped nuts, or a sprinkle of extra cinnamon if desired.

The apples and cinnamon give this oatmeal a delicious fall•inspired flavor. The honey adds a touch of sweetness. The almond milk makes it nice and creamy. This is a comforting and nutritious breakfast!

10. Breakfast Burrito:
Whole wheat tortilla,
scrambled eggs, avocado, salsa, cheese.

Ingredient:

- 4 large eggs
- 2 tbsp milk
- 1 tbsp butter
- 1/4 tsp salt
- 1/4 tsp black pepper
- 1 whole wheat tortilla
- 1/2 avocado, sliced
- 2 tbsp shredded cheddar or monterey jack cheese
- 2 tbsp salsa

Instructions:

1. In a small bowl, whisk together the eggs and milk. Season with salt and pepper.

2. Melt the butter in a nonstick skillet over medium heat. Pour in the egg mixture and cook, stirring occasionally, until the eggs are softly scrambled, about 2•3 minutes.

3. Warm the whole wheat tortilla according to package instructions, either in the microwave for 20•30 seconds or in a dry skillet for 30 seconds per side.

4. Lay the warmed tortilla on a flat surface. Spoon the scrambled eggs down the center. Top with sliced avocado, shredded cheese, and salsa.

5. Fold the bottom of the tortilla up over the filling, then fold in the sides and continue rolling up tightly into a burrito shape.

6. Serve the breakfast burrito immediately, while the eggs are still warm.

This breakfast burrito is packed with protein from the eggs, healthy fats from the avocado, and a kick of flavor from the salsa. The whole wheat tortilla makes it a more filling and nutritious start to the day.

11. Chia Pudding: Chia seeds, almond milk, honey, vanilla extract, berries.

Ingredient:

- 1/4 cup chia seeds
- 1 cup unsweetened almond milk
- 1 tbsp honey (or maple syrup)
- 1 tsp vanilla extract
- 1/2 cup mixed berries (such as blueberries, raspberries, strawberries)

Instructions:

1. In a medium bowl or mason jar, whisk together the chia seeds, almond milk, honey, and vanilla extract until well combined.

2. Cover and refrigerate for at least 4 hours, or overnight, stirring occasionally, until the chia seeds have thickened the mixture into a pudding•like consistency.

3. When ready to serve, give the chia pudding another stir. Top with the mixed berries.

4. Enjoy the chilled chia pudding straight from the fridge.

Optional Variations:

- Use different types of milk (dairy, coconut, etc.)
- Add a sprinkle of cinnamon or cocoa powder
- Top with chopped nuts, shredded coconut, or a drizzle of peanut butter

The chia seeds provide fiber, protein, and omega•3s. The almond milk and honey make it creamy and lightly sweetened. The vanilla adds warmth and the berries provide a fresh, fruity element. This make•ahead breakfast or snack is nutritious and delicious!

12. Ham and Cheese Omelette:
Eggs, ham, cheese, salt, pepper.

Ingredient:

- 3 eggs
- 1 tbsp milk or water
- 1/4 tsp salt
- 1/4 tsp black pepper
- 1 tbsp butter
- 2 slices diced ham
- 1/4 cup shredded cheddar or swiss cheese

Instructions:

1. Crack the eggs into a small bowl. Add the milk or water, salt, and pepper. Whisk the eggs until well blended.

2. Melt the butter in a small non•stick skillet over medium heat.

3. Pour the egg mixture into the hot skillet. As the eggs begin to set around the edges, use a spatula to gently push the cooked eggs towards the center, tilting the pan to allow the uncooked egg to flow to the edges.

4. When the eggs are mostly set but still a bit runny on top, sprinkle the diced ham and shredded cheese over half of the omelette.

5. Use the spatula to fold the unfilled half of the omelette over the half with the ham and cheese.

6. Cook for 1•2 minutes more, until the cheese is melted and the omelette is set.

7. Slide the omelette onto a plate and serve immediately.

The fluffy eggs, savory ham, and melty cheese make this a classic and satisfying breakfast omelette. Adjust the fillings to your liking • you can use different types of cheese or add other veggies as well.

13. Smoothie Bowl:
Frozen berries, banana, Greek yogurt, granola, honey.

Ingredient:

- 1 cup frozen mixed berries (such as blueberries, raspberries, strawberries)
- 1 ripe banana, frozen
- 1/2 cup plain Greek yogurt
- 1/4 cup unsweetened almond milk (or milk of your choice)
- 1 tbsp honey (or maple syrup)
- 1/4 cup granola
- Fresh berries for topping (optional)

Instructions:

1. In a high•powered blender, combine the frozen mixed berries, frozen banana, Greek yogurt, almond milk, and honey. Blend until smooth and creamy.

2. Pour the smoothie into a bowl.

3. Top the smoothie with the granola.

4. If desired, add a few fresh berries on top as well.

5. Serve the smoothie bowl immediately, with a spoon.

The frozen fruit and banana give the smoothie a thick, creamy texture. The Greek yogurt adds protein, while the honey provides natural sweetness. The granola topping adds a nice crunch.

You can customize the toppings to your liking • try other nuts, seeds, coconut flakes, or a drizzle of nut butter. This makes for a nutritious and satisfying breakfast or snack.

14. Egg Muffins:
Eggs, spinach, bell pepper, cheese, salt.

Ingredient:

- 8 large eggs
- 1/4 cup diced bell pepper (any color)
- 1/4 cup chopped fresh spinach
- 1/4 cup shredded cheddar or mozzarella cheese
- 1/4 tsp salt
- 1/4 tsp black pepper

Instructions:

1. Preheat your oven to 350°F (175°C). Grease a 12•cup muffin tin.

2. In a medium bowl, whisk the eggs. Stir in the diced bell pepper, chopped spinach, shredded cheese, salt, and pepper until well combined.

3. Divide the egg mixture evenly among the 12 muffin cups, filling each about 3/4 full.

4. Bake for 18•22 minutes, until the eggs are set and the muffins are lightly golden on top.

5. Allow the egg muffins to cool in the tin for 5 minutes before removing them.

6. Serve the egg muffins warm. They can also be refrigerated in an airtight container for up to 4 days.

These portable egg muffins are packed with protein, veggies, and melty cheese. They make a great grab•and•go breakfast or snack. You can customize the fillings to your liking • try adding diced ham, mushrooms, onions, or any other favorite omelet ingredients.

15. Protein Pancakes: Protein powder, oats, egg whites, banana, baking powder.

Ingredient:

- 1/2 cup rolled oats
- 1/4 cup vanilla protein powder
- 1/2 tsp baking powder
- 1/4 tsp salt
- 3 egg whites
- 1 ripe banana, mashed
- 2•3 tbsp unsweetened almond milk (or milk of your choice)

Toppings (optional):
- Fresh berries
- Maple syrup
- Nut butter
- Shredded coconut

Instructions:

1. In a medium bowl, combine the rolled oats, protein powder, baking powder, and salt. Stir to mix.

2. In a separate bowl, whisk the egg whites until frothy. Then mash the banana and stir it into the egg whites.

3. Pour the wet ingredients into the dry ingredients and stir just until combined. Add the almond milk 1 tablespoon at a time, until you reach a thick but pourable batter consistency.

4. Heat a nonstick skillet or griddle over medium heat. Lightly grease the surface.

5. Scoop the batter onto the hot surface, using about 1/4 cup for each pancake. Cook for 2•3 minutes per side, until golden brown.

6. Serve the protein pancakes warm, with your desired toppings.

These protein•packed pancakes are a great way to start the day. The oats, protein powder, and egg whites provide sustained energy. Top them with fresh fruit, a drizzle of maple syrup, or a spoonful of nut butter for added nutrition and flavor.

16. Green Smoothie:
Spinach, banana, almond milk, honey, ice.

Ingredient:

- 1 cup packed fresh spinach leaves
- 1 ripe banana, frozen
- 1 cup unsweetened almond milk
- 1 tbsp honey (or maple syrup)
- 1 cup ice cubes

Instructions:

1. In a high•powered blender, combine the spinach, frozen banana, almond milk, and honey.

2. Blend on high speed until the mixture is smooth and creamy, about 1•2 minutes.

3. Add the ice cubes and blend again until the smoothie is thick and frosty.

4. Pour the green smoothie into a glass and enjoy immediately.

Optional Variations:

- Use different greens like kale or swiss chard

- Add a scoop of protein powder

- Include other frozen fruit like pineapple or mango

- Use dairy milk or coconut milk instead of almond milk

- Top with chopped nuts, chia seeds, or shredded coconut

The spinach provides a boost of vitamins and minerals, while the banana and honey offer natural sweetness. The almond milk makes it nice and creamy. The ice gives it a refreshing, slushy texture.

This nutrient•dense green smoothie is a great way to start your day or enjoy as a healthy snack. It's easy to customize to your taste preferences.

17. Cottage Cheese and Fruit:
Cottage cheese, berries, honey, chia seeds, nuts.

Ingredient:

- 1 cup low•fat or full•fat cottage cheese
- 1 cup mixed berries (such as blueberries, raspberries, strawberries)
- 1 tbsp honey
- 1 tsp chia seeds
- 2 tbsp chopped nuts (such as almonds, walnuts, pecans)

Instructions:

1. In a parfait glass or bowl, layer half of the cottage cheese on the bottom.

2. Top the cottage cheese with half of the mixed berries.

3. Drizzle 1/2 tbsp of the honey over the berries.

4. Sprinkle 1/2 tsp of the chia seeds over the honey.

5. Repeat the layers, starting with the remaining cottage cheese, then the remaining berries, honey, and chia seeds.

6. Top the parfait with the chopped nuts.

7. Serve chilled or at room temperature.

Optional Variations:

- Use different types of fruit like mango, pineapple, or kiwi

- Add a sprinkle of cinnamon or vanilla extract

- Substitute Greek yogurt for the cottage cheese

- Use maple syrup or agave instead of honey

The cottage cheese provides protein, while the berries offer antioxidants and fiber. The honey adds natural sweetness, the chia seeds offer omega•3s, and the nuts provide a satisfying crunch. This makes for a nutritious and delicious breakfast or snack.

18. Veggie Breakfast Bowl:
Quinoa, avocado, cherry tomatoes, spinach, poached egg.

Ingredient:

- 1/2 cup cooked quinoa
- 1/2 avocado, sliced
- 1/2 cup cherry tomatoes, halved
- 1 cup fresh spinach leaves
- 1 poached egg
- 1 tbsp olive oil
- Salt and pepper to taste

Instructions:

1. Cook the quinoa according to package instructions. Set aside.

2. In a medium bowl, combine the cooked quinoa, sliced avocado, halved cherry tomatoes, and fresh spinach leaves.

3. Drizzle the veggie and quinoa mixture with the olive oil and season with salt and pepper.

4. Prepare a poached egg according to your preferred method.

5. Top the veggie breakfast bowl with the poached egg.

6. Serve the veggie breakfast bowl warm, with the runny yolk of the poached egg mixing in with the other ingredients.

Optional Additions:

- Sprinkle with crumbled feta or goat cheese

- Add a sprinkle of everything bagel seasoning

- Drizzle with a bit of balsamic glaze

- Include roasted sweet potato cubes

This nutrient•dense breakfast bowl is packed with protein, healthy fats, fiber, and vitamins. The combination of quinoa, avocado, tomatoes, spinach, and a poached egg makes for a satisfying and wholesome start to the day.

19. Almond Butter Toast: Whole grain bread, almond butter, banana, chia seeds, honey.

Ingredient:

- 2 slices whole grain bread
- 2 tbsp creamy almond butter
- 1 ripe banana, sliced
- 1 tsp chia seeds
- 1 tsp honey

Instructions:

1. Toast the two slices of whole grain bread until lightly golden brown.

2. Spread 1 tablespoon of almond butter evenly over each slice of toast.

3. Arrange the sliced banana over the almond butter.

4. Sprinkle the chia seeds over the banana slices.

5. Drizzle the honey over the top.

6. Serve the almond butter toast immediately.

Optional Variations:

- Use crunchy almond butter instead of creamy
- Add a sprinkle of cinnamon
- Swap the banana for other fruit like berries or apple slices
- Use peanut butter or another nut butter instead of almond butter
- Toast the bread in a skillet with a bit of butter for extra crispiness

This almond butter toast makes for a nutritious and satisfying breakfast or snack. The almond butter provides healthy fats and protein, the banana adds natural sweetness, the chia seeds offer fiber and omega•3s, and the honey gives it a touch of sweetness. The whole grain toast makes it a more filling and wholesome option.

20. Fruit Salad:
Mixed fruit, honey, lime juice, mint, chia seeds.

Ingredient:

- 2 cups mixed fruit (such as diced pineapple, mango, strawberries, blueberries, kiwi)
- 1 tbsp honey
- 1 tbsp fresh lime juice
- 1 tbsp chopped fresh mint leaves
- 1 tsp chia seeds

Instructions:

1. In a medium bowl, combine the mixed diced fruit.

2. Drizzle the honey and lime juice over the fruit and gently toss to coat.

3. Sprinkle the chopped mint leaves and chia seeds over the top.

4. Gently stir to incorporate the mint and chia seeds.

5. Cover and refrigerate the fruit salad for at least 30 minutes to allow the flavors to meld.

6. Serve the chilled fruit salad as a refreshing side dish or snack.

Optional Variations:

- Use different types of fruit like berries, citrus, grapes, etc.
- Add a splash of orange juice or a pinch of cinnamon
- Top with toasted nuts or shredded coconut
- Substitute agave or maple syrup for the honey

The combination of sweet and tart fruit, bright citrus, fragrant mint, and crunchy chia seeds makes this a delightful and nutritious fruit salad. The honey helps bring out the natural sweetness of the fruit. This is a great way to enjoy a variety of seasonal produce.

21. Grilled Chicken Salad: Grilled chicken, mixed greens, cherry tomatoes, cucumber, olive oil.

Ingredient:

- 4 boneless, skinless chicken breasts
- 1 tbsp olive oil, plus more for drizzling
- 1 tsp salt
- 1/2 tsp black pepper
- 5 oz mixed greens (such as spinach, arugula, kale)
- 1 cup cherry tomatoes, halved
- 1 cucumber, sliced
- 2 tbsp balsamic vinegar (or lemon juice)
- Salt and pepper to taste

Instructions:

1. Preheat grill or grill pan to medium•high heat.

2. Brush the chicken breasts with 1 tbsp of olive oil and season with salt and pepper.

3. Grill the chicken for 5•7 minutes per side, until cooked through. Allow to rest for 5 minutes, then slice or chop the chicken.

4. In a large salad bowl, combine the mixed greens, cherry tomatoes, and cucumber slices.

5. Add the grilled chicken to the salad.

6. Drizzle the salad with the balsamic vinegar (or lemon juice) and an additional 1•2 tbsp of olive oil. Season with salt and pepper to taste.

7. Toss the salad gently to coat the ingredients with the dressing. Serve the grilled chicken salad immediately.

Optional Additions:

- Top with crumbled feta or shredded cheddar cheese
- Add sliced avocado or roasted chickpeas
- Include toasted nuts or seeds for crunch

This grilled chicken salad is a simple yet satisfying meal. The combination of lean protein, fresh veggies, and a light dressing makes it a nutritious and flavorful option.

22. Turkey Wrap: Whole wheat tortilla, turkey slices, avocado, spinach, hummus.

Ingredient:

- 1 whole wheat tortilla
- 3•4 slices deli turkey
- 1/2 avocado, sliced
- 1 cup fresh spinach leaves
- 2 tbsp hummus

Instructions:

1. Lay the whole wheat tortilla flat on a clean surface.

2. Layer the turkey slices down the center of the tortilla.

3. Top the turkey with the sliced avocado and fresh spinach leaves.

4. Spread the hummus evenly over the spinach.

5. Fold the bottom of the tortilla up over the filling, then fold in the sides and continue rolling up tightly into a wrap shape.

6. Cut the wrap in half diagonally and serve immediately.

Optional Variations:

- Use a different type of deli meat like roast beef or ham

- Add shredded cheese, diced tomatoes, or sliced cucumber

- Swap the hummus for a different spread like cream cheese or pesto

- Use a flavored tortilla like spinach or tomato basil

This turkey wrap is a quick and easy lunch or snack option. The whole wheat tortilla provides complex carbs, the turkey offers lean protein, the avocado has healthy fats, and the spinach and hummus add extra nutrients. It's a well•balanced and portable meal.

23. Quinoa Salad: Quinoa, cherry tomatoes, cucumber, feta cheese, olive oil.

Ingredient:

- 1 cup cooked quinoa, cooled
- 1 cup cherry tomatoes, halved
- 1 cup diced cucumber
- 1/4 cup crumbled feta cheese
- 2 tbsp olive oil
- 1 tbsp red wine vinegar
- 1 tsp dried oregano
- 1/4 tsp salt
- 1/4 tsp black pepper

Instructions:

1. In a large bowl, combine the cooked and cooled quinoa, halved cherry tomatoes, diced cucumber, and crumbled feta cheese.

2. In a small bowl, whisk together the olive oil, red wine vinegar, dried oregano, salt, and black pepper.

3. Pour the dressing over the quinoa salad and toss gently to coat all the ingredients.

4. Refrigerate the quinoa salad for at least 30 minutes to allow the flavors to meld.

5. Serve chilled or at room temperature.

Optional Additions:

- Add diced red onion or sliced kalamata olives
- Toss in chopped fresh parsley or basil
- Use a different type of cheese like goat cheese or shredded mozzarella
- Add grilled or roasted chicken for extra protein

This quinoa salad is packed with nutrition from the whole grain quinoa, fresh veggies, and tangy feta cheese. The simple olive oil and vinegar dressing allows the flavors to shine. It makes a great side dish or light main course.

24. Chicken and Avocado Sandwich:
Whole grain bread, grilled chicken, avocado, lettuce, tomato.

Ingredient:

- 2 boneless, skinless chicken breasts
- 1 tbsp olive oil
- 1 tsp salt
- 1/2 tsp black pepper
- 4 slices whole grain bread
- 1 avocado, sliced
- 2 leaves lettuce
- 1 tomato, sliced

Instructions:

1. Preheat grill or grill pan to medium•high heat.

2. Brush the chicken breasts with the olive oil and season with salt and pepper.

3. Grill the chicken for 5•7 minutes per side, until cooked through. Allow to rest for 5 minutes, then slice or chop the chicken.

4. Toast the whole grain bread slices.

5. On each of the 4 toast slices, layer the following:

- Sliced grilled chicken
- Sliced avocado
- Lettuce leaves
- Tomato slices

6. Close the sandwiches with the remaining toast slices. Serve the chicken and avocado sandwiches immediately.

Optional Additions:

- Spread a thin layer of mayonnaise, mustard, or pesto on the bread
- Add a slice of cheese like cheddar or provolone
- Include crispy bacon or sautéed mushrooms
- Use a flavored bread like multigrain or sourdough

This chicken and avocado sandwich is a nutritious and satisfying meal. The whole grain bread, lean protein from the chicken, healthy fats from the avocado, and fresh veggies make it a well•balanced option. It's perfect for lunch or a light dinner.

25. Tuna Salad: Canned tuna, Greek yogurt, celery, red onion, lemon juice.

Ingredient:

- 2 (5 oz) cans tuna, drained
- 1/2 cup plain Greek yogurt
- 2 tbsp finely diced celery
- 2 tbsp finely diced red onion
- 1 tbsp fresh lemon juice
- 1/4 tsp salt
- 1/4 tsp black pepper

Instructions:

1. In a medium bowl, flake the drained tuna with a fork.

2. Add the Greek yogurt, diced celery, diced red onion, lemon juice, salt, and pepper. Stir to combine everything well.

3. Taste and adjust any seasonings as needed.

4. Serve the tuna salad on a bed of greens, in a sandwich, or with crackers.

Optional Variations:

- Add 1•2 tbsp of diced dill pickles or relish

- Stir in 1 tbsp of Dijon mustard

- Use plain low•fat or non•fat yogurt instead of Greek yogurt

- Add 1•2 tbsp of chopped fresh parsley or dill

- Substitute the lemon juice with red wine vinegar

This tuna salad is a healthier version that uses Greek yogurt instead of mayonnaise. The celery and onion add a nice crunch, while the lemon juice brightens up the flavors. It's a versatile dish that can be enjoyed in many different ways.

26. Caprese Salad: Tomatoes, mozzarella, basil, olive oil, balsamic vinegar.

Ingredient:

- 3 medium tomatoes, sliced
- 8 oz fresh mozzarella cheese, sliced
- 1/4 cup fresh basil leaves
- 2 tbsp olive oil
- 1 tbsp balsamic vinegar
- 1/4 tsp salt
- 1/4 tsp black pepper

Instructions:

1. Arrange the sliced tomatoes and mozzarella cheese on a serving platter or plate in an overlapping pattern.

2. Scatter the fresh basil leaves over the top.

3. Drizzle the olive oil and balsamic vinegar evenly over the salad.

4. Season with salt and black pepper.

5. Let the Caprese salad sit for 5•10 minutes to allow the flavors to meld.

6. Serve immediately, at room temperature.

Optional Variations:

- Use cherry or grape tomatoes, halved

- Add a drizzle of aged balsamic glaze

- Include a sprinkle of dried oregano or Italian seasoning

- Serve the Caprese salad on a bed of arugula or mixed greens. Skewer the tomato and mozzarella pieces for a fun presentation

The simple combination of juicy tomatoes, creamy mozzarella, and fragrant basil, dressed with high•quality olive oil and balsamic vinegar, makes this Caprese salad a classic Italian favorite. It's a refreshing and flavorful side dish or light main course.

27. Chicken Caesar Salad:
Romaine lettuce, grilled chicken, Caesar dressing, Parmesan, croutons.

Ingredient:

- 2 boneless, skinless chicken breasts
- 1 tbsp olive oil
- 1 tsp salt
- 1/2 tsp black pepper
- 6 cups chopped romaine lettuce
- 1/2 cup Caesar dressing
- 1/4 cup shredded Parmesan cheese
- 1/2 cup croutons

Instructions:

1. Preheat grill or grill pan to medium•high heat.

2. Brush the chicken breasts with the olive oil and season with salt and pepper.

3. Grill the chicken for 5•7 minutes per side, until cooked through. Allow to rest for 5 minutes, then slice or chop the chicken.

4. In a large salad bowl, combine the chopped romaine lettuce, grilled chicken, Caesar dressing, Parmesan cheese, and croutons.

5. Toss the salad gently to coat all the ingredients with the dressing.

6. Serve the Chicken Caesar Salad immediately.

Optional Variations:

- Use a store•bought Caesar dressing or make your own homemade version
- Add sliced hard•boiled eggs or anchovies for extra protein and flavor
- Include roasted garlic croutons or homemade seasoned croutons
- Sprinkle with toasted pine nuts or sunflower seeds
- Serve the salad in a hollowed•out romaine lettuce bowl

This classic Chicken Caesar Salad is a satisfying and flavorful meal. The grilled chicken provides lean protein, the romaine lettuce is packed with vitamins, and the Caesar dressing, Parmesan, and croutons add the signature Caesar flavors.

28. Veggie Wrap: Whole wheat tortilla, hummus, cucumber, bell pepper, spinach.

Ingredient:

- 1 whole wheat tortilla
- 2•3 tbsp hummus
- 1/4 cup sliced cucumber
- 1/4 cup sliced bell pepper (any color)
- 1 cup fresh spinach leaves
- 1 tbsp olive oil (optional)

Instructions:

1. Lay the whole wheat tortilla flat on a clean surface.

2. Spread the hummus evenly over the tortilla, leaving a 1•inch border.

3. Layer the sliced cucumber, bell pepper, and spinach leaves down the center of the tortilla.

4. If desired, drizzle the vegetables with a small amount of olive oil.

5. Fold the bottom of the tortilla up over the filling, then fold in the sides and continue rolling up tightly into a wrap shape.

6. Cut the wrap in half diagonally and serve immediately.

Optional Variations:

- Use a flavored hummus like roasted red pepper or garlic herb
- Add shredded carrots, sprouts, or sliced avocado
- Sprinkle with crumbled feta or shredded cheddar cheese
- Include a tablespoon of pesto or sun•dried tomato spread
- Use a spinach or tomato basil tortilla instead of whole wheat

This veggie wrap is a nutritious and portable meal or snack. The hummus provides protein and creaminess, while the fresh vegetables add crunch, flavor, and nutrients. It's a great way to pack in servings of veggies.

29. Egg Salad Sandwich: Whole grain bread, boiled eggs, Greek yogurt, mustard, lettuce.

Ingredient:

- 6 hard boiled eggs, peeled and chopped
- 1/4 cup plain Greek yogurt
- 1 tbsp Dijon mustard
- 1/4 tsp salt
- 1/4 tsp black pepper
- 4 slices whole grain bread
- 2 leaves lettuce

Instructions:

1. In a medium bowl, combine the chopped hard boiled eggs, Greek yogurt, Dijon mustard, salt, and pepper. Stir until well mixed.

2. Toast the whole grain bread slices.

3. Place a lettuce leaf on each of 2 toast slices.

4. Scoop the egg salad mixture evenly onto the lettuce•topped bread slices.

5. Top each sandwich with the remaining 2 toast slices.

6. Cut the egg salad sandwiches in half diagonally and serve.

Optional Variations:

- Add finely diced celery, onion, or pickle relish for extra crunch and flavor
- Use a flavored Greek yogurt like garlic and herb
- Swap the Dijon mustard for regular yellow mustard or spicy brown mustard
- Sprinkle the egg salad with paprika or chopped fresh dill
- Serve the egg salad on a bed of greens instead of bread

This egg salad sandwich is a nutritious and satisfying lunch option. The Greek yogurt provides creaminess while cutting down on mayonnaise, and the whole grain bread adds fiber. It's a classic comfort food with a healthy twist.

30. Avocado and Black Bean Salad:
Avocado, black beans, corn, cherry tomatoes, lime juice.

Ingredient:

- 1 ripe avocado, diced
- 1 (15 oz) can black beans, rinsed and drained
- 1 cup frozen corn kernels, thawed
- 1 cup cherry tomatoes, halved
- 2 tbsp fresh lime juice
- 1 tbsp olive oil
- 1/4 tsp salt
- 1/4 tsp black pepper
- 2 tbsp chopped fresh cilantro (optional)

Instructions:

1. In a large bowl, gently combine the diced avocado, black beans, thawed corn kernels, and halved cherry tomatoes.

2. Drizzle the lime juice and olive oil over the salad. Season with salt and pepper.

3. Toss the salad ingredients together until well coated with the dressing.

4. If desired, sprinkle the chopped fresh cilantro over the top.

5. Serve the avocado and black bean salad immediately or refrigerate until ready to serve.

Optional Variations:

- Add diced red onion or minced garlic for extra flavor
- Use a different type of bean like kidney or pinto beans
- Include diced jalapeño or a sprinkle of chili powder for a spicy kick
- Swap the corn for diced bell pepper or cucumber
- Serve the salad on a bed of mixed greens or with tortilla chips

This vibrant and flavorful avocado and black bean salad is packed with nutrients. The creamy avocado, protein•rich black beans, and fresh veggies make it a satisfying and versatile dish. It's great as a side salad or a light main course.

31. Shrimp Salad: Shrimp, mixed greens, avocado, cherry tomatoes, olive oil.

Ingredient:

- 1 lb cooked shrimp, peeled and deveined
- 5 oz mixed greens (such as spinach, arugula, kale)
- 1 avocado, diced
- 1 cup cherry tomatoes, halved
- 2 tbsp olive oil
- 1 tbsp lemon juice
- 1/4 tsp salt
- 1/4 tsp black pepper

Instructions:

1. In a large salad bowl, combine the cooked shrimp, mixed greens, diced avocado, and halved cherry tomatoes.

2. In a small bowl, whisk together the olive oil, lemon juice, salt, and black pepper to make the dressing.

3. Pour the dressing over the salad and toss gently to coat all the ingredients.

4. Serve the shrimp salad immediately.

Optional Variations:

- Add sliced cucumber or diced red onion

- Sprinkle with crumbled feta or shredded Parmesan cheese

- Include toasted nuts or seeds for extra crunch

- Drizzle with a balsamic glaze or vinaigrette instead of olive oil and lemon

- Use grilled or sautéed shrimp instead of cooked

This shrimp salad is a light and refreshing meal. The tender shrimp, creamy avocado, juicy tomatoes, and crisp greens make for a delicious and nutritious combination. The simple olive oil and lemon dressing allows the fresh flavors to shine.

32. Turkey and Cheese Sandwich:
Whole grain bread, turkey slices, cheese, lettuce, tomato.

Ingredient:

- 4 slices whole grain bread
- 4•6 slices deli turkey
- 2 slices cheese (cheddar, Swiss, provolone, etc.)
- 2 leaves lettuce
- 1 tomato, sliced

Instructions:

1. Toast the whole grain bread slices until lightly golden.

2. On one slice of toast, layer 2•3 slices of deli turkey.

3. Top the turkey with 1 slice of cheese.

4. Add a lettuce leaf and tomato slices.

5. Place another slice of toast on top to create a sandwich.

6. Repeat the process with the remaining ingredients to make a second sandwich.

7. Cut each sandwich in half diagonally and serve.

Optional Variations:

- Use a flavored bread like multigrain or sourdough

- Add a spread like mustard, mayo, or pesto

- Include other veggies like onion, cucumber, or avocado

- Swap the cheese for a different variety

- Toast the sandwich in a skillet with a bit of butter for a grilled effect

This classic turkey and cheese sandwich is a simple yet satisfying lunch option. The whole grain bread provides complex carbs, the turkey offers lean protein, and the cheese adds creaminess. The fresh lettuce and tomato provide crunch and juiciness. It's a well•balanced and portable meal.

33. Greek Salad:
Cucumber, cherry tomatoes, olives, feta cheese, olive oil.

Ingredient:

- 1 cucumber, diced
- 1 cup cherry tomatoes, halved
- 1/2 cup pitted kalamata olives, halved
- 1/2 cup crumbled feta cheese
- 2 tbsp olive oil
- 1 tbsp red wine vinegar
- 1 tsp dried oregano
- 1/4 tsp salt
- 1/4 tsp black pepper

Instructions:

1. In a large salad bowl, combine the diced cucumber, halved cherry tomatoes, halved kalamata olives, and crumbled feta cheese.

2. In a small bowl, whisk together the olive oil, red wine vinegar, dried oregano, salt, and black pepper.

3. Pour the dressing over the salad ingredients and toss gently to coat.

4. Let the Greek salad sit for 5•10 minutes to allow the flavors to meld.

5. Serve the Greek salad chilled or at room temperature.

Optional Variations:

- Add thinly sliced red onion or diced bell pepper
- Include cooked and cooled chickpeas or crumbled feta
- Drizzle with a bit of lemon juice for extra brightness
- Sprinkle with chopped fresh parsley or mint leaves
- Serve the salad on a bed of mixed greens

This classic Greek salad is full of fresh, vibrant flavors. The crisp cucumber, juicy tomatoes, briny olives, and creamy feta are a winning combination. The simple olive oil and vinegar dressing allows the natural flavors to shine.

34. Chicken and Veggie Stir•Fry:
Chicken breast, bell pepper, broccoli, soy sauce, olive oil.

Ingredient:

- 1 lb boneless, skinless chicken breasts, cut into 1•inch pieces
- 1 red bell pepper, sliced
- 2 cups broccoli florets
- 2 tbsp olive oil
- 2 tbsp low•sodium soy sauce
- 1 tsp minced garlic
- 1/4 tsp red pepper flakes (optional)
- Salt and pepper to taste
- Cooked brown rice, for serving (optional)

Instructions:

1. Heat the olive oil in a large skillet or wok over high heat.

2. Add the chicken pieces and stir•fry for 3•4 minutes until lightly browned.

3. Add the sliced bell pepper and broccoli florets. Stir•fry for 4•5 mInutes until the vegetables are tender•crisp.

4. Pour in the soy sauce and stir in the minced garlic and red pepper flakes (if using).

5. Continue to stir•fry for 1•2 minutes until the chicken is cooked through and the sauce has thickened slightly.

6. Season with salt and pepper to taste. Serve the chicken and veggie stir•fry immediately, over cooked brown rice if desired.

Optional Variations:

- Use a different protein like shrimp or tofu
- Add sliced mushrooms, snap peas, or baby corn
- Substitute the soy sauce with tamari or coconut aminos
- Garnish with chopped green onions or toasted sesame seeds
- Serve over cauliflower rice for a low•carb option

This chicken and veggie stir•fry is a quick, healthy, and flavorful meal. The combination of lean protein, fresh vegetables, and a savory sauce makes it a satisfying one•pan dish.

35. BLT Wrap: Whole wheat tortilla, bacon, lettuce, tomato, avocado.

Ingredient:

- 1 whole wheat tortilla
- 3•4 slices cooked bacon, crumbled
- 2•3 leaves romaine or green leaf lettuce
- 1 tomato, sliced
- 1/2 avocado, sliced
- 1 tbsp mayonnaise (optional)

Instructions:

1. Lay the whole wheat tortilla flat on a clean surface.

2. Spread the mayonnaise (if using) evenly over the tortilla, leaving a 1•inch border.

3. Layer the crumbled bacon, lettuce leaves, tomato slices, and avocado slices down the center of the tortilla.

4. Fold the bottom of the tortilla up over the filling, then fold in the sides and continue rolling up tightly into a wrap shape.

5. Cut the BLT wrap in half diagonally and serve.

Optional Variations:

- Use a flavored tortilla like spinach or sun•dried tomato

- Add a drizzle of balsamic glaze or hot sauce

- Include shredded cheddar or crumbled feta cheese

- Swap the bacon for grilled chicken or turkey

- Use mashed avocado instead of sliced

This BLT wrap is a delicious and portable twist on the classic bacon, lettuce, and tomato sandwich. The whole wheat tortilla provides a nutritious base, while the bacon, veggies, and avocado make it a satisfying meal. It's perfect for lunch or a light dinner.

36. Salmon Salad: Mixed greens, cooked salmon, avocado, cherry tomatoes, olive oil.

Ingredient:

- 5 oz mixed greens (such as spinach, arugula, kale)
- 6 oz cooked salmon, flaked
- 1 avocado, diced
- 1 cup cherry tomatoes, halved
- 2 tbsp olive oil
- 1 tbsp lemon juice
- 1/4 tsp salt
- 1/4 tsp black pepper

Instructions:

1. In a large salad bowl, combine the mixed greens, flaked cooked salmon, diced avocado, and halved cherry tomatoes.

2. In a small bowl, whisk together the olive oil, lemon juice, salt, and black pepper to make the dressing.

3. Pour the dressing over the salad and toss gently to coat all the ingredients.

4. Serve the salmon salad immediately.

Optional Variations:

- Top with toasted nuts or seeds for extra crunch
- Add sliced cucumber or red onion
- Sprinkle with crumbled feta or shredded Parmesan
- Drizzle with a balsamic glaze or vinaigrette
- Use grilled or pan•seared salmon instead of cooked

This salmon salad is a nutritious and satisfying meal. The omega•3 rich salmon, creamy avocado, juicy tomatoes, and crisp greens make for a delicious combination. The simple olive oil and lemon dressing allows the fresh flavors to shine.

37. Chicken Pita: Whole wheat pita, grilled chicken, hummus, cucumber, spinach.

Ingredient:

- 2 boneless, skinless chicken breasts
- 1 tbsp olive oil
- 1 tsp salt
- 1/2 tsp black pepper
- 2 whole wheat pita breads, halved
- 1/4 cup hummus
- 1/2 cucumber, sliced
- 1 cup fresh spinach leaves

Instructions:

1. Preheat grill or grill pan to medium•high heat.

2. Brush the chicken breasts with the olive oil and season with salt and pepper.

3. Grill the chicken for 5•7 minutes per side, until cooked through. Allow to rest for 5 minutes, then slice or chop the chicken.

4. Spread 2 tbsp of hummus inside each pita half.

5. Layer the sliced grilled chicken, cucumber slices, and fresh spinach leaves into the pita halves. Serve the chicken pitas immediately.

Optional Variations:

- Use a flavored hummus like roasted red pepper or garlic
- Add diced tomatoes, shredded carrots, or sliced red onion
- Sprinkle with crumbled feta or shredded cheddar cheese
- Drizzle with a bit of olive oil or balsamic glaze
- Substitute the spinach with other greens like arugula or romaine

This chicken pita is a nutritious and portable meal. The whole wheat pita provides complex carbs, the grilled chicken offers lean protein, the hummus adds creaminess, and the fresh veggies provide crunch and nutrients. It's a well•balanced and flavorful option.

38. Veggie Sandwich: Whole grain bread, hummus, avocado, cucumber, spinach.

Ingredient:

- 4 slices whole grain bread
- 1/4 cup hummus
- 1/2 avocado, sliced
- 1/2 cucumber, sliced
- 1 cup fresh spinach leaves
- Salt and pepper to taste

Instructions:

1. Toast the whole grain bread slices until lightly golden.

2. Spread 1•2 tablespoons of hummus evenly over 2 of the toast slices.

3. Layer the avocado slices, cucumber slices, and fresh spinach leaves over the hummus.

4. Season with a pinch of salt and pepper.

5. Top with the remaining 2 toast slices to create the sandwiches.

6. Cut each sandwich in half diagonally and serve.

Optional Variations:

- Use a flavored hummus like roasted red pepper or garlic
- Add sliced tomatoes, shredded carrots, or sprouts
- Include a slice of cheese like cheddar or provolone
- Drizzle with a bit of olive oil or balsamic glaze
- Toast the sandwich in a skillet with a small amount of butter

This veggie sandwich is a nutritious and satisfying meatless option. The whole grain bread provides complex carbs, the hummus offers protein and creaminess, the avocado has healthy fats, and the fresh veggies add crunch and nutrients. It's a delicious and filling lunch or snack.

39. Steak Salad: Mixed greens, grilled steak, cherry tomatoes, avocado, olive oil.

Ingredient:

- 8 oz flank steak or sirloin steak
- 1 tbsp olive oil
- 1 tsp salt
- 1/4 tsp salt
- 1/4 tsp black pepper

- 1/2 tsp black pepper
- 5 oz mixed greens (such as spinach, arugula, kale)
- 1 cup cherry tomatoes, halved
- 1 avocado, diced
- 2 tbsp olive oil
- 1 tbsp balsamic vinegar

Instructions:

1. Preheat grill or grill pan to medium•high heat.

2. Brush the steak with 1 tbsp of olive oil and season with 1 tsp salt and 1/2 tsp black pepper.

3. Grill the steak for 4•6 minutes per side, until it reaches your desired doneness. Allow to rest for 5 minutes, then slice or chop the steak.

4. In a large salad bowl, combine the mixed greens, halved cherry tomatoes, and diced avocado.

5. In a small bowl, whisk together the 2 tbsp olive oil, balsamic vinegar, 1/4 tsp salt, and 1/4 tsp black pepper to make the dressing.

6. Add the sliced or chopped grilled steak to the salad. Drizzle the dressing over the top and toss gently to coat. Serve the steak salad immediately.

Optional Variations:

- Top with crumbled feta or shredded Parmesan cheese
- Include roasted vegetables like bell peppers or mushrooms
- Swap the balsamic vinegar for red wine vinegar or lemon juice
- Use a different type of steak like flank, skirt, or ribeye

This steak salad is a hearty and satisfying meal. The tender grilled steak, fresh greens, juicy tomatoes, and creamy avocado make for a delicious and nutritious combination. The simple olive oil and balsamic dressing complements the flavors perfectly.

40. Chickpea Salad: Chickpeas, cherry tomatoes, cucumber, feta cheese, olive oil.

Ingredient:

- 1 (15 oz) can chickpeas, drained and rinsed
- 1 cup cherry tomatoes, halved
- 1 cucumber, diced
- 1/2 cup crumbled feta cheese
- 2 tbsp olive oil
- 1 tbsp lemon juice
- Salt and pepper to taste

Instructions:

1. In a large bowl, combine the drained and rinsed chickpeas, halved cherry tomatoes, diced cucumber, and crumbled feta cheese.

2. Drizzle the olive oil and lemon juice over the salad and toss gently to coat.

3. Season with salt and pepper to taste.

4. Refrigerate for at least 30 minutes to allow the flavors to meld.

5. Serve chilled or at room temperature.

Enjoy your fresh and flavorful Chickpea Salad!

41. Grilled Salmon:
Salmon fillet, lemon, olive oil, salt, pepper.

Ingredient:

- 4 salmon fillets (about 6 oz each)
- 2 tbsp olive oil
- 1 lemon, cut into wedges
- Salt and pepper to taste

Instructions:

1. Preheat your grill to medium•high heat.

2. Pat the salmon fillets dry with paper towels and brush both sides with the olive oil. Season generously with salt and pepper.

3. Place the salmon fillets skin•side down on the preheated grill grates. Grill for 4•6 minutes per side, or until the salmon flakes easily with a fork and reaches your desired doneness.

4. Transfer the grilled salmon to a serving platter. Serve immediately with the lemon wedges on the side.

Optional Variations:

- Brush the salmon with a bit of honey or maple syrup before grilling for a sweet glaze.

- Sprinkle the salmon with chopped fresh herbs like dill, parsley, or chives.

- Serve the grilled salmon over a bed of greens or with roasted vegetables.

Enjoy your delicious and simple Grilled Salmon!

42. Chicken and Broccoli:
Chicken breast, broccoli, olive oil, garlic, soy sauce.

Ingredient:

- 1 lb boneless, skinless chicken breasts, cut into 1•inch pieces
- 2 cups broccoli florets
- 2 tbsp olive oil
- 3 cloves garlic, minced
- 1 tsp grated ginger
- 2 tbsp low•sodium soy sauce
- 1 tbsp rice vinegar
- 1 tsp sesame oil
- Salt and pepper to taste
- Cooked rice, for serving

Instructions:

1. In a large skillet or wok, heat the olive oil over medium•high heat. Add the chicken and cook for 5•7 minutes, stirring occasionally, until the chicken is lightly browned.

2. Add the broccoli, garlic, and ginger to the skillet. Cook for 3•4 minutes, stirring frequently, until the broccoli is tender•crisp.

3. In a small bowl, whisk together the soy sauce, rice vinegar, and sesame oil. Pour the sauce into the skillet and toss everything together to coat.

4. Season with salt and pepper to taste.

5. Serve the chicken and broccoli over cooked rice.

Enjoy your delicious and healthy Chicken and Broccoli!

43. Beef Stir-Fry: Beef strips, bell pepper, broccoli, soy sauce, olive oil.

Ingredient:

- 1 lb beef strips or thinly sliced beef (such as flank steak or sirloin)
- 1 bell pepper, sliced
- 2 cups broccoli florets
- 2 tbsp soy sauce
- 1 tbsp olive oil
- 2 cloves garlic, minced
- Salt and pepper to taste
- Cooked rice, for serving

Instructions:

1. In a large skillet or wok, heat the olive oil over high heat.

2. Add the beef strips and stir•fry for 2•3 minutes, until the beef is lightly browned on the outside but still pink inside. Transfer the beef to a plate.

3. Add the bell pepper and broccoli to the skillet. Stir•fry for 3•4 minutes, until the vegetables are tender•crisp.

4. Return the beef to the skillet along with the soy sauce and garlic. Stir•fry for 1•2 minutes, until everything is heated through.

5. Season with salt and pepper to taste.

6. Serve the beef stir•fry immediately over cooked rice.

Tips:

- Slice the beef against the grain for the most tender texture.
- Feel free to add other vegetables like mushrooms, snap peas, or carrots.
- Adjust the soy sauce amount to your taste preference.

Enjoy your quick and easy Beef Stir•Fry!

44. Baked Cod:
Cod fillet, lemon, olive oil, salt, pepper.

Ingredient:

- 4 cod fillets (about 6 oz each)
- 2 tbsp olive oil
- 1 lemon, cut into wedges
- Salt and pepper to taste

Instructions:

1. Preheat your oven to 400°F (200°C).

2. Pat the cod fillets dry with paper towels and place them on a baking sheet lined with parchment paper or foil.

3. Brush the top of the cod fillets with the olive oil and season generously with salt and pepper.

4. Bake the cod in the preheated oven for 12•15 minutes, or until the fish flakes easily with a fork and is opaque throughout.

5. Serve the baked cod immediately, with the lemon wedges on the side. The lemon juice can be squeezed over the fish just before eating.

Optional Variations:

- Sprinkle the cod with chopped fresh herbs like parsley, dill, or thyme before baking.
- Top the cod with breadcrumbs or Parmesan cheese for a crispy topping.
- Serve the baked cod over a bed of roasted vegetables or a salad.

Enjoy your simple and delicious Baked Cod!

45. Turkey Meatballs: Ground turkey, egg, breadcrumbs, Parmesan, marinara sauce.

Ingredient:

- 1 lb ground turkey
- 1 egg
- 1/2 cup breadcrumbs
- 1/4 cup grated Parmesan cheese
- 2 cloves garlic, minced
- 1 tsp dried oregano
- 1/2 tsp salt
- 1/4 tsp black pepper
- 2 cups marinara sauce

Instructions:

1. Preheat your oven to 400°F (200°C).

2. In a large bowl, combine the ground turkey, egg, breadcrumbs, Parmesan, garlic, oregano, salt, and pepper. Mix well until all the ingredients are evenly distributed.

3. Roll the mixture into 1•inch meatballs and place them on a baking sheet lined with parchment paper.

4. Bake the meatballs in the preheated oven for 18•20 minutes, or until they are cooked through and lightly browned.

5. In a saucepan, heat the marinara sauce over medium heat.

6. Add the baked meatballs to the marinara sauce and gently stir to coat them.

7. Serve the turkey meatballs and marinara sauce over cooked pasta, zucchini noodles, or with a side of garlic bread.

Optional Variations:

- Add finely chopped onion or bell pepper to the meatball mixture.
- Use a combination of ground turkey and ground beef for a richer flavor.
- Bake the meatballs on a wire rack set over a baking sheet for even browning.

46. Chicken Fajitas:
Chicken breast, bell pepper, onion, tortillas, salsa.

Ingredient:

- 1 lb boneless, skinless chicken breasts, sliced into thin strips
- 1 red bell pepper, sliced
- 1 green bell pepper, sliced
- 1 onion, sliced
- 2 tbsp olive oil
- 2 tsp chili powder
- 1 tsp cumin
- 1 tsp garlic powder
- Salt and pepper to taste
- 8•10 small tortillas (corn or flour)
- Salsa, for serving
- Optional toppings:
 guacamole, sour cream, shredded cheese

Instructions:

1. In a large skillet or wok, heat the olive oil over medium•high heat.

2. Add the chicken strips, bell peppers, and onion to the skillet. Season with the chili powder, cumin, garlic powder, salt, and pepper.

3. Stir•fry the mixture for 8•10 minutes, or until the chicken is cooked through and the vegetables are tender•crisp.

4. Warm the tortillas according to package instructions.

5. To serve, place some of the chicken and vegetable mixture into the center of each tortilla. Top with your desired toppings, such as salsa, guacamole, sour cream, and shredded cheese. Fold the tortillas and enjoy your Chicken Fajitas!

Tips:

- You can use a mix of different colored bell peppers for more visual appeal.
- Marinate the chicken in a mixture of lime juice, olive oil, and spices for added flavor.
- Serve the fajitas with rice and beans for a more complete meal

47. Shrimp Tacos:
Shrimp, tortillas, avocado, salsa, lime.

Ingredient:

- 1 lb shrimp, peeled and deveined
- 2 tbsp olive oil
- 1 tsp chili powder
- 1 tsp cumin
- Salt and pepper to taste
- 8•10 small tortillas (corn or flour)
- 1 avocado, sliced
- Salsa, for serving
- Lime wedges, for serving

Instructions:

1. In a large skillet, heat the olive oil over medium•high heat.

2. Season the shrimp with the chili powder, cumin, salt, and pepper. Add the seasoned shrimp to the hot skillet and cook for 2•3 minutes per side, until the shrimp are opaque and cooked through.

3. Remove the shrimp from the skillet and set aside.

4. Warm the tortillas according to package instructions.

5. To assemble the tacos, place a few pieces of shrimp in the center of each tortilla. Top with sliced avocado and a spoonful of salsa. Serve the shrimp tacos immediately, with lime wedges on the side for squeezing over the top.

Optional Toppings:

- Shredded cabbage or lettuce
- Crumbled queso fresco or shredded cheese
- Chopped cilantro
- Sour cream

Tips:

- You can use a mix of different colored salsas for more flavor and visual appeal.
- Marinate the shrimp in a mixture of lime juice, olive oil, and spices for added flavor.
- Serve the shrimp tacos with a side of rice and beans for a more complete meal.

48. Stuffed Peppers: Bell peppers, ground turkey, quinoa, marinara sauce, cheese.

Ingredient:

- 4 bell peppers (any color), halved and seeded
- 1 lb ground turkey
- 1 cup cooked quinoa
- 1 cup marinara sauce
- 1/2 cup shredded mozzarella cheese
- 2 cloves garlic, minced
- 1 tsp dried oregano
- Salt and pepper to taste

Instructions:

1. Preheat your oven to 375°F (190°C).

2. In a large bowl, combine the ground turkey, cooked quinoa, 1/2 cup of the marinara sauce, garlic, oregano, salt, and pepper. Mix well until all the ingredients are evenly distributed.

3. Arrange the bell pepper halves in a baking dish or on a rimmed baking sheet.

4. Spoon the turkey•quinoa mixture evenly into the bell pepper halves.

5. Pour the remaining 1/2 cup of marinara sauce over the stuffed peppers.

6. Sprinkle the shredded mozzarella cheese over the top.

7. Bake the stuffed peppers in the preheated oven for 30•35 minutes, or until the peppers are tender and the filling is heated through.

8. Serve the stuffed peppers hot, garnished with additional fresh herbs if desired.

Optional Variations:

- Use a combination of ground turkey and ground beef for the filling.
- Add diced onion, mushrooms, or other vegetables to the filling.
- Sprinkle the top with breadcrumbs or Parmesan cheese for a crispy topping.
- Serve the stuffed peppers over a bed of rice or quinoa.

49. Pork Chops:
Pork chops, olive oil, garlic, rosemary, salt.

Ingredient:

- 4 boneless pork chops (about 1•inch thick)
- 2 tbsp olive oil
- 3 cloves garlic, minced
- 2 tsp fresh rosemary, chopped (or 1 tsp dried rosemary)
- 1 tsp salt
- 1/2 tsp black pepper

Instructions:

1. Pat the pork chops dry with paper towels and season them all over with the salt and pepper.

2. In a large skillet or cast•iron pan, heat the olive oil over medium•high heat.

3. Add the pork chops to the hot pan and cook for 4•5 minutes per side, or until they are golden brown and cooked through. The internal temperature should reach 145°F (63°C).

4. During the last minute of cooking, add the minced garlic and chopped rosemary to the pan. Stir and cook until fragrant.

5. Transfer the pork chops to a plate and let them rest for 5 minutes before serving.

Optional Variations:

- Marinate the pork chops in a mixture of olive oil, lemon juice, garlic, and herbs for added flavor.

- Bake the pork chops in the oven at 400°F (200°C) for 20•25 minutes, flipping halfway through.

- Serve the pork chops with roasted vegetables, mashed potatoes, or a fresh salad.

Enjoy your delicious Pork Chops!

50. Zucchini Noodles with Pesto:
Zucchini, pesto, cherry tomatoes, Parmesan, olive oil.

Ingredient:

- 4 medium zucchinis, spiralized or julienned into noodles
- 1/2 cup basil pesto
- 1 cup cherry tomatoes, halved
- 1/4 cup grated Parmesan cheese
- 2 tbsp olive oil
- Salt and pepper to taste

Instructions:

1. In a large skillet or wok, heat the olive oil over medium heat.

2. Add the zucchini noodles to the skillet and cook for 2•3 minutes, just until they start to soften but are still al dente. Be careful not to overcook them.

3. Remove the skillet from the heat and add the basil pesto. Toss the noodles to coat them evenly with the pesto.

4. Stir in the halved cherry tomatoes and grated Parmesan cheese. Season with salt and pepper to taste.

5. Serve the zucchini noodles with pesto immediately, garnished with additional Parmesan cheese or fresh basil leaves if desired.

Optional Variations:

- Use a different type of pesto, such as sun•dried tomato or arugula pesto.

- Add grilled or sautéed chicken or shrimp for a protein•packed meal.

- Sprinkle toasted pine nuts or sliced almonds over the top for extra crunch.

- Serve the zucchini noodles with pesto cold, as a refreshing summer salad.

Enjoy your delicious and healthy Zucchini Noodles with Pesto!

51. Baked Chicken:
Chicken breast, lemon, garlic, olive oil, thyme.

Ingredient:

- 4 boneless, skinless chicken breasts
- 2 tbsp olive oil
- 2 cloves garlic, minced
- 1 lemon, zested and juiced
- 1 tsp dried thyme
- Salt and pepper to taste

Instructions:

1. Preheat your oven to 400°F (200°C).

2. In a small bowl, combine the olive oil, minced garlic, lemon zest, lemon juice, and dried thyme. Season with salt and pepper.

3. Place the chicken breasts in a baking dish or on a rimmed baking sheet. Pour the garlic•lemon mixture over the chicken, making sure to evenly coat the chicken.

4. Bake the chicken in the preheated oven for 25•30 minutes, or until the chicken is cooked through and reaches an internal temperature of 165°F (74°C).

5. Remove the baked chicken from the oven and let it rest for 5 minutes before serving.

Optional Variations:

• Sprinkle the chicken with grated Parmesan cheese or breadcrumbs for a crispy topping.

• Add sliced lemon or fresh thyme sprigs to the baking dish for extra flavor.

• Serve the baked chicken with roasted vegetables or a fresh salad.

• Marinate the chicken in the garlic•lemon mixture for 30 minutes to 1 hour before baking for more intense flavor.

Enjoy your delicious Baked Chicken!

52. Tuna Steak:
Tuna steak, soy sauce, ginger, garlic, olive oil.

Ingredient:

- 4 tuna steaks (about 6 oz each)
- 2 tbsp soy sauce
- 1 tbsp grated fresh ginger
- 2 cloves garlic, minced
- 1 tbsp olive oil
- Salt and pepper to taste

Instructions:

1. In a shallow dish, whisk together the soy sauce, grated ginger, and minced garlic.

2. Add the tuna steaks to the dish and turn to coat both sides with the soy sauce mixture. Cover and let marinate for 30 minutes to 1 hour in the refrigerator.

3. Heat the olive oil in a large skillet or grill pan over medium•high heat.

4. Remove the tuna steaks from the marinade and season both sides with salt and pepper.

5. Carefully add the tuna steaks to the hot skillet or grill pan. Cook for 2•3 minutes per side, or until the tuna is cooked to your desired doneness. Avoid overcooking the tuna, as it is best served rare or medium•rare.

6. Transfer the seared tuna steaks to a plate and let them rest for 5 minutes before serving.

Optional Variations:

- Brush the tuna steaks with a teriyaki or honey•soy glaze during the last minute of cooking.

- Serve the tuna steaks over a bed of greens or with roasted vegetables.

- Garnish the tuna with sliced green onions, sesame seeds, or a drizzle of sesame oil.

Enjoy your delicious Tuna Steak!

53. Spaghetti Squash with Marinara: Spaghetti squash, marinara sauce, Parmesan, olive oil, basil.

Ingredient:

- 1 medium spaghetti squash
- 2 cups marinara sauce
- 1/4 cup grated Parmesan cheese
- 2 tbsp olive oil
- 2 cloves garlic, minced
- 1/4 cup fresh basil leaves, chopped
- Salt and pepper to taste

Instructions:

1. Preheat your oven to 400°F (200°C).

2. Cut the spaghetti squash in half lengthwise and scoop out the seeds. Place the squash halves cut•side up on a baking sheet.

3. Bake the spaghetti squash in the preheated oven for 40•50 minutes, or until it's tender and easily shreds with a fork.

4. Remove the spaghetti squash from the oven and let it cool slightly. Using a fork, gently shred the flesh of the squash into spaghetti•like strands.

5. In a large skillet, heat the olive oil over medium heat. Add the minced garlic and cook for 1 minute, until fragrant.

6. Add the shredded spaghetti squash to the skillet and toss to coat with the garlic oil. Cook for 2•3 minutes, stirring occasionally.

7. Pour the marinara sauce over the spaghetti squash and stir to combine. Heat through, about 2•3 minutes.

8. Remove the skillet from the heat and stir in the grated Parmesan cheese and chopped fresh basil.

9. Season with salt and pepper to taste. Serve the spaghetti squash with marinara immediately.

54. Lamb Chops:
Lamb chops, olive oil, garlic, rosemary, salt.

Ingredient:

- 4 lamb chops (about 1•inch thick)
- 2 tbsp olive oil
- 3 cloves garlic, minced
- 2 tsp fresh rosemary, chopped (or 1 tsp dried rosemary)
- 1 tsp salt
- 1/2 tsp black pepper

Instructions:

1. Pat the lamb chops dry with paper towels and season them all over with the salt and pepper.

2. In a large skillet or cast•iron pan, heat the olive oil over medium•high heat.

3. Add the lamb chops to the hot pan and cook for 3•4 minutes per side, or until they are nicely browned on the outside and cooked to your desired doneness. For medium•rare, the internal temperature should reach 130•135°F (54•57°C).

4. During the last minute of cooking, add the minced garlic and chopped rosemary to the pan. Stir and cook until fragrant.

5. Transfer the lamb chops to a plate and let them rest for 5 minutes before serving.

Optional Variations:

- Marinate the lamb chops in a mixture of olive oil, lemon juice, garlic, and herbs for added flavor.

- Broil the lamb chops in the oven for 4•6 minutes per side, or until cooked to your liking.

- Serve the lamb chops with roasted potatoes, a fresh salad, or sautéed vegetables.

- Garnish the lamb chops with additional fresh rosemary or a drizzle of balsamic glaze.

Enjoy your delicious Lamb Chops!

55. Grilled Shrimp Skewers:
Shrimp, olive oil, garlic, lemon, paprika.

Ingredient:

- 1 lb large shrimp, peeled and deveined
- 2 tbsp olive oil
- 3 cloves garlic, minced
- 1 lemon, zested and juiced
- 1 tsp paprika
- 1/2 tsp salt
- 1/4 tsp black pepper
- Wooden or metal skewers

Instructions:

1. In a large bowl, combine the olive oil, minced garlic, lemon zest, lemon juice, paprika, salt, and pepper. Add the shrimp and toss to coat evenly.

2. If using wooden skewers, soak them in water for 30 minutes to prevent them from burning on the grill.

3. Thread the marinated shrimp onto the skewers, leaving a small space between each shrimp.

4. Preheat your grill to medium•high heat.

5. Grill the shrimp skewers for 2•3 minutes per side, or until the shrimp are opaque and cooked through.

6. Serve the grilled shrimp skewers immediately, garnished with additional lemon wedges if desired.

Optional Variations:

- Add chopped fresh herbs, such as parsley, cilantro, or basil, to the marinade.
- Use a combination of shrimp and cubed chicken or pork on the skewers.
- Brush the shrimp skewers with a glaze made from honey, soy sauce, and Dijon mustard during the last minute of grilling.
- Serve the grilled shrimp skewers over a bed of rice or with a fresh salad.

56. Turkey Chili: Ground turkey, kidney beans, diced tomatoes, onion, chili powder.

Ingredient:

- 1 lb ground turkey
- 1 onion, diced
- 3 cloves garlic, minced
- 2 cans (15 oz each) kidney beans, drained and rinsed
- 1 can (28 oz) diced tomatoes
- 2 tbsp chili powder
- 1 tsp cumin
- 1 tsp oregano
- 1/2 tsp salt
- 1/4 tsp black pepper
- Shredded cheese, sour cream, and chopped cilantro for serving (optional)

Instructions:

1. In a large pot or Dutch oven, cook the ground turkey over medium•high heat, breaking it up with a wooden spoon, until it's no longer pink, about 5•7 minutes.

2. Add the diced onion and minced garlic to the pot. Cook for 2•3 minutes, until the onion is translucent.

3. Stir in the kidney beans, diced tomatoes, chili powder, cumin, oregano, salt, and pepper. Bring the mixture to a simmer.

4. Reduce the heat to medium•low and let the chili simmer for 20•25 minutes, stirring occasionally, until the flavors have melded and the chili has thickened.

5. Taste and adjust the seasoning as needed.

6. Serve the turkey chili hot, topped with shredded cheese, sour cream, and chopped cilantro, if desired.

Optional Variations:

- Add diced bell peppers or jalapeños for extra flavor and heat.
- Use a combination of ground turkey and ground beef for a richer chili.
- Stir in a can of corn or diced sweet potatoes for extra vegetables.
- Serve the chili over cooked rice or with cornbread on the side

57. Chicken Kabobs:
Chicken breast, bell pepper, onion, olive oil, garlic.

Ingredient:

- 1 lb boneless, skinless chicken breasts, cut into 1•inch cubes
- 1 red bell pepper, cut into 1•inch pieces
- 1 green bell pepper, cut into 1•inch pieces
- 1 onion, cut into 1•inch pieces
- 2 tbsp olive oil
- 3 cloves garlic, minced
- 1 tsp dried oregano
- 1/2 tsp salt
- 1/4 tsp black pepper
- Wooden or metal skewers

Instructions:

1. In a large bowl, combine the chicken cubes, bell pepper pieces, and onion pieces.

2. In a small bowl, whisk together the olive oil, minced garlic, dried oregano, salt, and black pepper.

3. Pour the marinade over the chicken and vegetable mixture and toss to coat everything evenly.

4. If using wooden skewers, soak them in water for 30 minutes to prevent them from burning on the grill.

5. Thread the marinated chicken and vegetables onto the skewers, alternating the ingredients. Preheat your grill to medium•high heat.

6. Grill the chicken kabobs for 12•15 minutes, turning occasionally, until the chicken is cooked through and the vegetables are tender. Serve the grilled chicken kabobs immediately.

Optional Variations:

- Marinate the chicken and vegetables in a mixture of lemon juice, soy sauce, and honey for added flavor.
- Use a variety of vegetables, such as zucchini, mushrooms, or cherry tomatoes.
- Brush the kabobs with a glaze made from barbecue sauce or teriyaki sauce during the last few minutes of grilling.

58. Stuffed Zucchini: Zucchini, ground turkey, marinara sauce, cheese, olive oil.

Ingredient:

- 4 medium zucchinis, halved lengthwise
- 1 lb ground turkey
- 1 cup marinara sauce
- 1/2 cup shredded mozzarella cheese
- 2 tbsp olive oil
- 2 cloves garlic, minced
- 1 tsp dried oregano
- 1/2 tsp salt
- 1/4 tsp black pepper

Instructions:

1. Preheat your oven to 375°F (190°C).

2. Using a spoon or melon baller, scoop out the flesh from the center of each zucchini half, leaving a 1/4•inch border. Chop the scooped•out zucchini flesh.

3. In a large skillet, heat the olive oil over medium heat. Add the chopped zucchini flesh, ground turkey, minced garlic, oregano, salt, and pepper. Cook, breaking up the turkey with a wooden spoon, until the turkey is cooked through and the zucchini is tender, about 8•10 minutes.

4. Remove the skillet from the heat and stir in 1/2 cup of the marinara sauce.

5. Arrange the zucchini halves in a baking dish. Spoon the turkey•zucchini mixture into the hollowed•out zucchini halves.

6. Top the stuffed zucchini halves with the remaining 1/2 cup of marinara sauce and the shredded mozzarella cheese.

7. Bake the stuffed zucchini in the preheated oven for 20•25 minutes, or until the zucchini is tender and the cheese is melted and bubbly. Serve the Stuffed Zucchini hot, garnished with additional fresh herbs if desired.

Optional Variations:
- Use a combination of ground turkey and ground beef for the filling.
- Add diced onion, bell pepper, or mushrooms to the filling.
- Sprinkle the top with breadcrumbs or Parmesan cheese for a crispy topping.
- Serve the Stuffed Zucchini over a bed of pasta or with a side salad.

59. Steak and Asparagus:
Steak, asparagus, olive oil, garlic, salt.

Ingredient:

- 1 lb flank steak or skirt steak, cut into thin strips
- 1 lb asparagus, trimmed and cut into 2•inch pieces
- 2 tbsp olive oil
- 3 cloves garlic, minced
- 1 tsp salt
- 1/4 tsp black pepper

Instructions:

1. In a large skillet or wok, heat the olive oil over medium•high heat.

2. Add the steak strips to the hot pan and cook for 2•3 minutes, stirring occasionally, until the steak is lightly browned on the outside but still pink inside.

3. Add the asparagus pieces and minced garlic to the pan. Continue to cook for 3•4 minutes, stirring frequently, until the asparagus is tender•crisp and the steak is cooked to your desired doneness.

4. Season the steak and asparagus with the salt and black pepper. Toss everything together to coat evenly.

5. Serve the Steak and Asparagus immediately, while hot.

Optional Variations:

- Marinate the steak in a mixture of soy sauce, rice vinegar, and sesame oil before cooking for added flavor.
- Add sliced mushrooms or diced onions to the pan for extra vegetables.
- Serve the Steak and Asparagus over a bed of cooked rice or quinoa.
- Garnish the dish with chopped fresh parsley or green onions.

Tips:

- Use a high•heat cooking method, such as a hot skillet or wok, to ensure the steak and asparagus cook quickly and remain tender.
- Slice the steak against the grain for the most tender texture.
- Adjust the cooking time for the asparagus based on your desired level of doneness.

60. Baked Tilapia:
Tilapia fillet, lemon, olive oil, garlic, dill.

Ingredient:

- 4 tilapia fillets (about 6 oz each)
- 2 tbsp olive oil
- 2 cloves garlic, minced
- 1 lemon, cut into wedges
- 2 tbsp chopped fresh dill (or 1 tsp dried dill)
- Salt and pepper to taste

Instructions:

1. Preheat your oven to 400°F (200°C).

2. Place the tilapia fillets in a baking dish or on a rimmed baking sheet. Drizzle the olive oil over the fillets and use your hands or a brush to evenly coat them.

3. Sprinkle the minced garlic and chopped fresh dill (or dried dill) over the top of the fillets. Season with salt and pepper to taste.

4. Bake the tilapia in the preheated oven for 15•18 minutes, or until the fish flakes easily with a fork and is opaque throughout.

5. Serve the baked tilapia immediately, with the lemon wedges on the side. The lemon juice can be squeezed over the fish just before eating.

Optional Variations:

- Top the tilapia with a breadcrumb or Parmesan cheese topping for a crispy crust.
- Substitute the dill with other fresh herbs, such as parsley, basil, or thyme.
- Serve the baked tilapia over a bed of roasted vegetables or a fresh salad.
- Drizzle the baked tilapia with a lemon•butter sauce or a pesto sauce.

Enjoy your delicious Baked Tilapia!

61. Apple Slices with Peanut Butter:
Apple, peanut butter, cinnamon, chia seeds, honey.

Ingredient:

- 2 apples, cored and sliced
- 1/4 cup peanut butter
- 1 tsp ground cinnamon
- 1 tbsp chia seeds
- 1 tbsp honey (optional)

Instructions:

1. Wash and core the apples, then slice them into thin wedges or rounds.

2. Arrange the apple slices on a serving plate or platter.

3. In a small bowl, mix together the peanut butter, ground cinnamon, and chia seeds until well combined.

4. Spoon or drizzle the peanut butter mixture over the apple slices, making sure to cover them evenly.

5. If desired, drizzle a small amount of honey over the top of the peanut butter•coated apple slices.

Optional Variations:

- Use almond butter or another nut butter instead of peanut butter.
- Sprinkle the apple slices with a pinch of sea salt for a sweet and salty flavor.
- Add a sprinkle of granola or chopped nuts for extra crunch.
- Serve the apple slices with a side of Greek yogurt for a protein•packed snack.
- Use a variety of apple types, such as Gala, Honeycrisp, or Fuji, for different flavors and textures.

Enjoy your delicious and healthy Apple Slices with Peanut Butter!

62. Trail Mix: Almonds, cashews, dried cranberries, dark chocolate chips, sunflower seeds.

Ingredient:

- 1 cup raw almonds
- 1 cup raw cashews
- 1/2 cup dried cranberries
- 1/2 cup dark chocolate chips
- 1/4 cup roasted and salted sunflower seeds

Instructions:

1. In a large bowl, combine the almonds, cashews, dried cranberries, dark chocolate chips, and sunflower seeds.

2. Stir the ingredients together until they are evenly distributed.

3. Transfer the trail mix to an airtight container or resealable bag for storage.

Optional Variations:

- Use a variety of nuts, such as pecans, walnuts, or pumpkin seeds.

- Add other dried fruits, like raisins, apricots, or cherries.

- Include a small amount of unsweetened coconut flakes or toasted coconut.

- Sprinkle in a pinch of ground cinnamon or a dash of cayenne pepper for a spicy twist.

- Use milk chocolate or white chocolate chips instead of dark chocolate.

- Roast the nuts and seeds before adding them to the mix for a deeper flavor.

Tips:

- Store the trail mix in a cool, dry place, away from direct sunlight, to keep the ingredients fresh.
- Adjust the ratios of the ingredients to suit your personal taste preferences.
- This trail mix makes a great snack on its own or can be added to yogurt, oatmeal, or baked goods.

63. Hummus and Veggies: Hummus, carrot sticks, cucumber, bell pepper, cherry tomatoes.

Ingredient:

- 1 cup store•bought or homemade hummus
- 1 cup carrot sticks
- 1 cup cucumber slices
- 1 cup bell pepper strips (any color)
- 1 cup cherry tomatoes

Instructions:

1. Arrange the hummus in a small bowl or on a plate.

2. Arrange the carrot sticks, cucumber slices, bell pepper strips, and cherry tomatoes around the hummus, creating a colorful vegetable platter.

Optional Variations:

- Use a variety of hummus flavors, such as roasted red pepper, garlic, or sun•dried tomato.

- Include other crunchy vegetables like celery sticks, radish slices, or jicama sticks.

- Add a sprinkle of paprika, za'atar, or chopped fresh herbs on top of the hummus.

- Serve the hummus and veggies with pita bread, whole•grain crackers, or tortilla chips for dipping.

- For a heartier snack, top the hummus with a drizzle of olive oil, a sprinkle of feta cheese, and a few kalamata olives.

Tips:

- Choose a high•quality, creamy hummus for the best flavor and texture.

- Wash and prepare the vegetables in advance for a quick and easy snack.

- Adjust the vegetable quantities based on your personal preferences and the number of people you're serving. Serve the hummus and veggies chilled or at room temperature.

64. Greek Yogurt with Honey:
Greek yogurt, honey, walnuts, chia seeds, berries.

Ingredient:

- 1 cup plain Greek yogurt
- 2 tbsp honey
- 2 tbsp chopped walnuts
- 1 tbsp chia seeds
- 1/2 cup mixed berries (such as blueberries, raspberries, and/or strawberries)

Instructions:

1. In a medium bowl, scoop the Greek yogurt and drizzle the honey over the top.

2. Sprinkle the chopped walnuts and chia seeds over the yogurt and honey.

3. Top with the mixed berries. Gently stir the ingredients together until they are well combined.

Optional Variations:

- Use a flavored Greek yogurt, such as vanilla or honey, instead of plain.

- Substitute the walnuts with other nuts, such as almonds, pecans, or pistachios.

- Add a sprinkle of granola or a drizzle of peanut butter for extra crunch and flavor.

- Use a variety of fresh or frozen berries, such as blackberries, blueberries, raspberries, and strawberries.

- Sprinkle a pinch of cinnamon or a squeeze of lemon juice over the top. Serve the Greek yogurt parfait•style in a tall glass or jar for a more elegant presentation.

Tips:

- Use high•quality, full•fat Greek yogurt for a richer, creamier texture. Adjust the amount of honey to your desired sweetness level.

- Prepare the Greek yogurt with honey and toppings just before serving for the freshest flavor.

65. Protein Balls: Oats, peanut butter, honey, protein powder, dark chocolate chips.

Ingredient:

- 1 cup old•fashioned oats
- 1/2 cup peanut butter (or other nut butter)
- 1/4 cup honey
- 2 scoops (about 1/2 cup) vanilla protein powder
- 2 tbsp dark chocolate chips

Instructions:

1. In a medium bowl, combine the oats, peanut butter, and honey. Mix until well incorporated.

2. Add the protein powder and stir until the mixture is evenly combined and forms a sticky dough.

3. Fold in the dark chocolate chips.

4. Using a small cookie scoop or your hands, form the mixture into 1•inch balls.

5. Place the protein balls on a parchment•lined baking sheet or plate.

6. Refrigerate the protein balls for at least 30 minutes to allow them to firm up. Store the protein balls in an airtight container in the refrigerator for up to 1 week.

Optional Variations:
- Use a different type of nut butter, such as almond butter or cashew butter.
- Add a pinch of cinnamon or a splash of vanilla extract for extra flavor.
- Roll the protein balls in shredded coconut, chopped nuts, or cocoa powder for a coated exterior.
- Substitute the dark chocolate chips with other mix•ins, like dried fruit, seeds, or mini chocolate chips.
- Use a combination of different protein powders, such as whey and plant•based.

Tips:

- Adjust the amount of honey or nut butter to achieve the desired consistency and sweetness.
- Chill the protein balls before serving for a firmer texture.

66. Fruit and Nut Bars:
Dates, almonds, cashews, dried cranberries, honey.

Ingredient:

- 1 cup pitted Medjool dates
- 1 cup raw almonds
- 1 cup raw cashews
- 1/2 cup dried cranberries
- 2 tbsp honey

Instructions:

1. Line an 8x8 inch baking pan with parchment paper, leaving some overhang on the sides for easy removal.

2. In a food processor, pulse the pitted Medjool dates until they form a sticky, paste•like consistency.

3. Add the raw almonds and cashews to the food processor and pulse until the nuts are finely chopped and well combined with the date paste.

4. Transfer the nut and date mixture to the prepared baking pan. Use your hands or the back of a spoon to firmly press the mixture into an even layer.

5. Sprinkle the dried cranberries evenly over the top of the nut and date mixture.

6. Drizzle the honey over the cranberries, using the back of a spoon to gently spread it around.

7. Cover the pan with plastic wrap or foil and refrigerate for at least 2 hours, or until the bars are firm.

8. Once chilled, use the parchment paper overhang to lift the bars out of the pan. Cut into 12 equal bars.

9. Store the Fruit and Nut Bars in an airtight container in the refrigerator for up to 1 week.

67. Veggie Chips:
Kale, olive oil, salt, pepper, paprika.

Ingredient:

- 1 bunch kale, stems removed and leaves torn into bite•sized pieces
- 2 tbsp olive oil
- 1 tsp salt
- 1/2 tsp black pepper
- 1/2 tsp paprika

Instructions:

1. Preheat your oven to 350°F (175°C).

2. In a large bowl, toss the kale leaves with the olive oil, salt, black pepper, and paprika until the leaves are evenly coated.

3. Spread the kale leaves in a single layer on two large baking sheets lined with parchment paper.

4. Bake the kale chips in the preheated oven for 12•15 minutes, flipping them halfway through, until they are crispy and lightly browned.

5. Remove the kale chips from the oven and let them cool completely on the baking sheets.

Optional Variations:

- Use other types of vegetables, such as thinly sliced zucchini, beets, or sweet potatoes, to make a variety of veggie chips.

- Experiment with different seasonings, such as garlic powder, onion powder, cayenne pepper, or Italian herbs.

- Drizzle the kale or vegetable chips with a bit of honey or maple syrup for a sweet and savory flavor.

- Sprinkle the chips with grated Parmesan cheese or a blend of shredded cheeses.

- Serve the veggie chips with a dipping sauce, such as ranch, hummus, or tzatziki.

68. Edamame:
Edamame, sea salt, lemon juice, olive oil, pepper.

Ingredient:

- 1 lb frozen edamame, in the pod
- 1 tbsp sea salt
- 1 tbsp lemon juice
- 1 tsp olive oil
- 1/4 tsp black pepper

Instructions:

1. Bring a large pot of water to a boil over high heat.

2. Add the frozen edamame pods to the boiling water and cook for 5•7 minutes, or until the pods are tender and bright green.

3. Drain the cooked edamame in a colander and transfer them to a serving bowl.

4. Sprinkle the sea salt over the hot edamame and toss to coat.

5. Drizzle the lemon juice and olive oil over the edamame and season with the black pepper.

6. Serve the edamame warm, with the pods still intact, allowing your guests to pop the beans out of the pods and enjoy.

Optional Variations:

- Use a combination of sea salt and toasted sesame seeds for a nutty flavor.

- Add a pinch of crushed red pepper flakes for a spicy kick.

- Substitute the lemon juice with a splash of soy sauce or rice vinegar.

- Serve the edamame chilled, rather than warm, for a refreshing snack.

- Offer small bowls or plates for guests to discard the empty edamame pods.

69. Cottage Cheese with Pineapple:
Cottage cheese, pineapple, honey, chia seeds, almonds.

Ingredient:

- 1 cup low•fat or non•fat cottage cheese
- 1/2 cup diced fresh pineapple or canned pineapple tidbits, drained
- 1 tsp honey (optional)
- Mint leaves for garnish (optional)

Instructions:

1. In a small bowl, combine the cottage cheese and diced pineapple.

2. If desired, drizzle the honey over the top and stir gently to combine.

3. Garnish with fresh mint leaves, if using.

4. Serve chilled or at room temperature.

This makes a refreshing and healthy snack or light dessert. The sweetness of the pineapple pairs nicely with the creamy cottage cheese. You can adjust the amount of pineapple to your taste preference. Enjoy!

70. Banana Chips:
Bananas, lemon juice, cinnamon, coconut oil, honey.

Ingredient:

- 3 ripe but firm bananas, sliced into 1/8•inch thick rounds
- 1 tbsp lemon juice
- 1 tsp ground cinnamon
- 1 tbsp coconut oil, melted
- 1 tbsp honey (optional)

Instructions:

1. Preheat your oven to 135°F (57°C). Line two baking sheets with parchment paper.

2. In a large bowl, toss the banana slices with the lemon juice until well coated. This will help prevent browning.

3. Arrange the banana slices in a single layer on the prepared baking sheets. Make sure the slices are not overlapping.

4. In a small bowl, mix together the ground cinnamon, melted coconut oil, and honey (if using).

5. Drizzle the cinnamon•coconut oil mixture over the banana slices, using a pastry brush or your fingers to lightly coat each slice.

6. Bake the banana chips in the preheated oven for 2•3 hours, flipping the slices halfway through, until they are crispy and golden brown.

7. Turn off the oven and leave the banana chips inside for an additional 1•2 hours, or until completely dried and crispy.

8. Remove the banana chips from the oven and let them cool completely on the baking sheets. Store the homemade banana chips in an airtight container at room temperature for up to 1 week.

Optional Variations:

- Sprinkle the banana chips with a pinch of sea salt or a dash of cayenne pepper for a savory twist.
- Dip the banana chips in melted dark chocolate or drizzle with melted white chocolate.
- Use a dehydrator instead of an oven for a more consistent and efficient drying process.

71. Pumpkin Seeds:
Pumpkin seeds, olive oil, salt, pepper, paprika.

Ingredient:

- 1 cup raw pumpkin seeds (also called pepitas)
- 1 tbsp olive oil
- 1/2 tsp salt
- 1/4 tsp black pepper
- 1/4 tsp paprika

Instructions:

1. Preheat your oven to 325°F (165°C).

2. In a small bowl, toss the raw pumpkin seeds with the olive oil, salt, pepper, and paprika until the seeds are evenly coated.

3. Spread the seasoned pumpkin seeds in a single layer on a baking sheet.

4. Roast for 15•20 minutes, stirring halfway, until the seeds are lightly golden brown and crispy.

5. Remove from the oven and let cool slightly before serving.

The roasted pumpkin seeds make a great snack or topping for salads, soups, and other dishes. The olive oil, salt, pepper, and paprika add a tasty seasoning to the seeds. You can adjust the amounts of the seasonings to your taste preference.

72. Guacamole and Veggies:
Avocado, lime juice, garlic, salt, bell pepper.

Ingredient:

- 3 ripe avocados, pitted and diced
- 2 tbsp fresh lime juice
- 2 cloves garlic, minced
- 1/2 tsp salt
- 1 bell pepper, sliced into strips (any color)
- 1 cup baby carrots
- 1 cup cherry tomatoes, halved

Instructions:

1. In a medium bowl, mash the diced avocados with a fork or potato masher until they reach your desired consistency.

2. Stir in the lime juice, minced garlic, and salt. Mix well to combine.

3. Arrange the guacamole in a serving bowl or on a plate.

4. Surround the guacamole with the sliced bell pepper strips, baby carrots, and halved cherry tomatoes.

Optional Variations:

- Add diced onion, chopped cilantro, or diced jalapeño to the guacamole for extra flavor.
- Use a combination of different colored bell peppers for a more vibrant presentation.
- Serve the guacamole and veggies with whole•grain crackers, pita chips, or tortilla chips for dipping.
- Garnish the guacamole with a sprinkle of paprika or chili powder.
- Offer a small bowl of lime wedges for guests to squeeze over the guacamole.

Tips:

- Choose ripe, creamy avocados for the best guacamole texture.
- Mash the avocados just before serving to prevent them from browning.
- Adjust the amount of lime juice and salt to suit your taste preferences.
- Prepare the vegetable crudités in advance and store them in the refrigerator until ready to serve.
- Serve the guacamole and veggies chilled or at room temperature.

73. Cheese and Crackers: Cheese, whole grain crackers, apple slices, almonds, honey.

Ingredient:

- 8 oz assorted cheese (such as cheddar, gouda, brie, or blue cheese), sliced or cubed
- 1 cup whole grain crackers
- 1 apple, sliced
- 1/2 cup raw almonds
- 2 tbsp honey (optional)

Instructions:

1. Arrange the sliced or cubed cheese on a serving platter or board.

2. Place the whole grain crackers around the cheese.

3. Add the apple slices and raw almonds to the platter.

4. If desired, drizzle a small amount of honey over the cheese and apple slices.

Optional Variations:

- Use a variety of cheese types, such as sharp cheddar, creamy brie, and crumbly blue cheese.
- Substitute the apple slices with other fresh fruit, like grapes, pears, or figs.
- Add a small bowl of olives, dried apricots, or fig jam to the platter.
- Sprinkle the almonds with a pinch of cinnamon or sea salt.
- Serve the cheese and crackers with a small knife or cheese spreader.

Tips:

- Choose a mix of hard, soft, and semi•soft cheeses for a variety of textures and flavors.
- Slice or cube the cheese ahead of time for easy serving.
- Arrange the items on the platter in a visually appealing way, with the cheese as the focal point.
- Serve the cheese and crackers at room temperature for the best flavor and texture.
- Provide a small plate or napkins for guests to use when assembling their bites

74. Smoothie Popsicles: Greek yogurt, mixed berries, honey, almond milk, chia seeds.

Ingredient:

- 1 cup plain Greek yogurt
- 1 cup mixed berries (such as strawberries, blueberries, raspberries)
- 2 tbsp honey
- 1/2 cup unsweetened almond milk
- 1 tbsp chia seeds

Instructions:

1. In a blender, combine the Greek yogurt, mixed berries, honey, almond milk, and chia seeds. Blend until smooth.

2. Carefully pour the smoothie mixture into popsicle molds, leaving a little room at the top for expansion.

3. Insert popsicle sticks into the molds.

4. Freeze the popsicles for at least 4 hours, or until completely frozen.

5. To remove the popsicles from the molds, run the molds under warm water for a few seconds, then gently pull the popsicles out.

The Greek yogurt provides protein, the berries add antioxidants and natural sweetness, the honey is a natural sweetener, the almond milk adds creaminess, and the chia seeds provide fiber and omega•3s.

These smoothie popsicles make a refreshing and healthy treat, perfect for hot summer days. You can experiment with different fruit combinations as well.

Enjoy your homemade Smoothie Popsicles!

75. Almond Butter Energy Bites: Oats, almond butter, honey, chia seeds, dark chocolate chips.

Ingredient:

- 1 cup old•fashioned oats
- 1/2 cup creamy almond butter
- 1/4 cup honey
- 2 tbsp chia seeds
- 2 tbsp dark chocolate chips

Instructions:

1. In a medium bowl, stir together the oats, almond butter, honey, and chia seeds until well combined.

2. Fold in the dark chocolate chips.

3. Using a tablespoon or small cookie scoop, form the mixture into bite•sized balls.

4. Place the energy bites on a parchment•lined baking sheet or plate.

5. Refrigerate for at least 30 minutes to allow the bites to firm up.

6. Store the energy bites in an airtight container in the refrigerator for up to 1 week.

The oats provide complex carbs and fiber, the almond butter adds healthy fats and protein, the honey is a natural sweetener, the chia seeds offer omega•3s and fiber, and the dark chocolate chips provide a touch of antioxidants and richness.

These Almond Butter Energy Bites make a great portable snack or pre•workout fuel. You can adjust the amounts of the ingredients to suit your taste preferences.

Enjoy your homemade Almond Butter Energy Bites!

76. Roasted Chickpeas:
Chickpeas, olive oil, salt, pepper, paprika.

Ingredient:

- 1 (15 oz) can chickpeas (garbanzo beans), drained and rinsed
- 1 tbsp olive oil
- 1/2 tsp salt
- 1/4 tsp black pepper
- 1/4 tsp paprika

Instructions:

1. Preheat your oven to 400°F (200°C).

2. Pat the drained and rinsed chickpeas dry with paper towels or a clean kitchen towel. This helps them get crispy when roasted.

3. In a medium bowl, toss the chickpeas with the olive oil, salt, pepper, and paprika until the chickpeas are evenly coated.

4. Spread the seasoned chickpeas in a single layer on a baking sheet.

5. Roast for 20•25 minutes, stirring halfway, until the chickpeas are crispy and lightly browned.

6. Remove from the oven and let cool slightly before serving.

The roasted chickpeas make a great snack or topping for salads, soups, and other dishes. The olive oil, salt, pepper, and paprika add a tasty seasoning to the chickpeas. You can adjust the amounts of the seasonings to your taste preference.

Enjoy your homemade roasted chickpeas!

77. Frozen Yogurt Bark:
Greek yogurt, honey, mixed berries, granola, chia seeds.

Ingredient:

- 2 cups plain Greek yogurt
- 2 tbsp honey
- 1 cup mixed berries (such as blueberries, raspberries, blackberries)
- 1/2 cup granola
- 1 tbsp chia seeds

Instructions:

1. Line a baking sheet with parchment paper or a silicone baking mat.

2. In a medium bowl, stir together the Greek yogurt and honey until well combined.

3. Spread the yogurt mixture evenly onto the prepared baking sheet, creating a thin, even layer.

4. Sprinkle the mixed berries, granola, and chia seeds over the top of the yogurt.

5. Gently press the toppings into the yogurt to help them adhere.

6. Place the baking sheet in the freezer and freeze for at least 4 hours, or until the yogurt bark is completely frozen.

7. Once frozen, break or cut the yogurt bark into irregular pieces.

8. Store the frozen yogurt bark in an airtight container in the freezer for up to 2 months.

The Greek yogurt provides protein, the honey adds natural sweetness, the berries offer antioxidants, the granola adds crunch, and the chia seeds contribute fiber and omega•3s.

This Frozen Yogurt Bark makes a refreshing and healthy snack or dessert. You can customize the toppings to your liking, such as using different types of berries, nuts, or seeds.

Enjoy your homemade Frozen Yogurt Bark!

78. Apple Nachos: Apple slices, peanut butter, dark chocolate chips, coconut flakes, almonds.

Ingredient:

- 2 large apples, cored and sliced into thin wedges
- 1/4 cup creamy peanut butter
- 2 tbsp dark chocolate chips
- 2 tbsp unsweetened shredded coconut
- 2 tbsp chopped almonds

Instructions:

1. Arrange the apple slices in a single layer on a large plate or platter to create your "nachos".

2. In a small microwave•safe bowl, heat the peanut butter for 20•30 seconds, just until softened and drizzle•able.

3. Drizzle the warm peanut butter over the apple slices.

4. Sprinkle the dark chocolate chips, shredded coconut, and chopped almonds evenly over the top.

5. Serve immediately, while the peanut butter is still warm and drizzly.

The crisp, juicy apple slices act as the "chips" for this healthy and delicious snack. The peanut butter provides protein and healthy fats, the dark chocolate chips add richness, the coconut flakes add texture, and the almonds offer a nice crunch.

You can customize the toppings to your liking • try using different nut butters, seeds, dried fruit, or even a drizzle of honey or caramel sauce.

These Apple Nachos make a fun, easy, and nutritious snack or light dessert. Enjoy!

79. Fruit Skewers:
Mixed fruit, honey, lime juice, mint, chia seeds.

Ingredient:

- 1 cup mixed fruit (such as pineapple, strawberries, grapes, melon, kiwi)
- 2 tbsp honey
- 1 tbsp fresh lime juice
- 1 tbsp fresh mint leaves, chopped
- 1 tsp chia seeds

Instructions:

1. Wash and prepare the fruit by cutting it into bite•sized pieces.

2. Thread the fruit pieces onto wooden or metal skewers, alternating the different types of fruit.

3. In a small bowl, whisk together the honey and lime juice until well combined.

4. Drizzle the honey•lime mixture over the fruit skewers, making sure to coat them evenly.

5. Sprinkle the chopped mint leaves and chia seeds over the top of the fruit skewers.

6. Refrigerate the fruit skewers for at least 30 minutes to allow the flavors to meld.

7. Serve the chilled fruit skewers as a refreshing and healthy snack or dessert.

The combination of sweet and tangy flavors from the honey, lime, and fresh fruit is delightful. The mint adds a refreshing herbal note, while the chia seeds provide a nutritional boost.

You can use any variety of fresh, seasonal fruits that you prefer. The skewers make for a visually appealing and portable snack.

Enjoy your homemade Fruit Skewers!

80. Cucumber Sandwiches: Cucumber, cream cheese, smoked salmon, dill, lemon juice.

Ingredient:

- 1 English cucumber, thinly sliced
- 4 oz cream cheese, softened
- 4 oz smoked salmon, thinly sliced
- 2 tbsp fresh dill, chopped
- 1 tbsp lemon juice

Instructions:

1. In a small bowl, mix together the softened cream cheese, chopped dill, and lemon juice until well combined.

2. Lay the cucumber slices on a clean work surface. Spread a thin layer of the cream cheese mixture onto each slice.

3. Top half of the cucumber slices with a piece of smoked salmon.

4. Place the remaining cucumber slices, cream cheese side down, on top of the salmon to create little "sandwiches".

5. Chill the cucumber sandwiches in the refrigerator for at least 30 minutes before serving to allow the flavors to meld.

6. Serve chilled or at room temperature.

The cool, crisp cucumber provides a nice contrast to the creamy cheese and salty smoked salmon. The dill and lemon juice add freshness. These cucumber sandwiches make a great light appetizer or snack.

You can adjust the amounts of the ingredients to your taste preferences. You can also try using different types of smoked fish or herbs.

Enjoy your homemade Cucumber Sandwiches!

81. Chocolate Avocado Mousse: Avocado, cocoa powder, honey, vanilla extract, almond milk.

Ingredient:

- 2 ripe avocados, pitted and flesh scooped out
- 1/4 cup unsweetened cocoa powder
- 1/4 cup honey (or maple syrup)
- 1 tsp vanilla extract
- 1/4 cup unsweetened almond milk

Instructions:

1. In a food processor or high•powered blender, combine the avocado flesh, cocoa powder, honey, and vanilla extract. Blend until smooth and creamy, scraping down the sides as needed.

2. With the motor running, slowly pour in the almond milk and continue blending until the mixture is silky and well•incorporated.

3. Taste and adjust sweetness if desired, adding a bit more honey or maple syrup.

4. Transfer the chocolate avocado mousse to individual serving dishes or one larger serving bowl.

5. Refrigerate for at least 2 hours, or until chilled and set.

6. Serve chilled, garnished with fresh berries, shaved dark chocolate, or a dusting of cocoa powder if desired.

The avocado provides a rich, creamy base, while the cocoa powder gives it a deep chocolate flavor. The honey (or maple syrup) sweetens it up, and the almond milk helps achieve a light, airy texture.

This Chocolate Avocado Mousse is a healthy, dairy•free, and decadent dessert or snack. The avocado also adds beneficial fats, fiber, and nutrients.

Enjoy your homemade Chocolate Avocado Mousse!

82. Berry Crumble:
Mixed berries, oats, honey, almond flour, coconut oil.

Ingredient:

For the Filling:
- 3 cups mixed berries (such as blueberries, raspberries, blackberries)
- 2 tbsp honey
- 1 tbsp cornstarch

For the Crumble Topping:
- 1 cup old•fashioned oats
- 1/2 cup almond flour
- 3 tbsp honey
- 3 tbsp coconut oil, melted

Instructions:

1. Preheat your oven to 375°F (190°C).

For **the** Filling:

2. In a medium bowl, gently toss the mixed berries with the honey and cornstarch until the berries are evenly coated.
3. Transfer the berry mixture to a baking dish.

For the Crumble Topping:

4. In a separate bowl, combine the oats, almond flour, honey, and melted coconut oil. Mix until the mixture resembles coarse crumbs.
5. Sprinkle the crumble topping evenly over the berry filling.

Baking:

6. Bake the berry crumble for 25•30 minutes, or until the topping is golden brown and the filling is bubbling.

7. Allow the crumble to cool for 10•15 minutes before serving.

Serve the warm berry crumble on its own or with a scoop of vanilla ice cream or whipped cream. The sweet, juicy berries paired with the crunchy, nutty topping make for a delicious and satisfying dessert.

83. Banana Ice Cream: Bananas, almond milk, vanilla extract, cocoa powder, honey.

Ingredient:

- 3 ripe bananas, sliced and frozen
- 1/2 cup unsweetened almond milk
- 1 tsp vanilla extract
- 2 tbsp unsweetened cocoa powder
- 1 tbsp honey (optional)

Instructions:

1. In a high•powered blender or food processor, combine the frozen banana slices, almond milk, and vanilla extract. Blend until smooth and creamy, scraping down the sides as needed.

2. Add the cocoa powder and honey (if using) and blend again until fully incorporated.

3. Serve the banana ice cream immediately for a soft, soft•serve consistency.

4. For a firmer, scoopable ice cream, transfer the mixture to a freezer•safe container and freeze for 2•3 hours, stirring every 30 minutes, until desired consistency is reached.

The frozen bananas provide the base for this creamy, guilt•free ice cream. The almond milk adds creaminess, the vanilla enhances the flavor, the cocoa powder gives it a chocolatey taste, and the honey provides natural sweetness (if desired).

This banana ice cream is dairy•free, vegan, and requires no special equipment beyond a blender or food processor. It's a healthy, delicious treat that's perfect for hot summer days.

Enjoy your homemade Banana Ice Cream!

84. Chia Seed Pudding: Chia seeds, almond milk, honey, vanilla extract, berries.

Ingredient:

- 1/4 cup chia seeds
- 1 cup unsweetened almond milk
- 2 tbsp honey
- 1 tsp vanilla extract
- 1 cup mixed berries (such as blueberries, raspberries, strawberries)

Instructions:

1. In a medium bowl, whisk together the chia seeds, almond milk, honey, and vanilla extract until well combined.

2. Cover the bowl and refrigerate for at least 2 hours, or up to 24 hours, stirring occasionally, until the mixture has thickened to a pudding•like consistency.

3. Once the chia pudding has set, divide it evenly between 4 serving bowls or jars.

4. Top each serving with 1/4 cup of the mixed berries.

5. Serve chilled.

The chia seeds swell up in the almond milk, creating a thick, creamy pudding. The honey provides natural sweetness, while the vanilla extract enhances the flavor. The fresh berries add a burst of color, flavor, and antioxidants.

This Chia Seed Pudding is a nutritious, make•ahead breakfast or snack. It's high in fiber, protein, and healthy omega•3s from the chia seeds.

You can customize the toppings with other fresh fruit, nuts, seeds, or a drizzle of nut butter.

Enjoy your homemade Chia Seed Pudding!

85. Apple Crisp:
Apples, oats, honey, cinnamon, almond flour.

Ingredient:

For the Filling:
• 4 cups peeled, cored, and sliced apples (about 4•5 medium apples)
• 2 tbsp honey
• 1 tsp ground cinnamon

For the Topping:
• 1 cup old•fashioned oats
• 1/2 cup almond flour
• 2 tbsp honey
• 2 tbsp coconut oil, melted
• 1/2 tsp ground cinnamon

Instructions:

1. Preheat your oven to 350°F (175°C).

For the Filling:

2. In a large bowl, toss the sliced apples with the 2 tbsp of honey and 1 tsp of cinnamon until the apples are evenly coated.
3. Transfer the apple mixture to a baking dish.

For the Topping:

4. In a separate bowl, combine the oats, almond flour, 2 tbsp of honey, melted coconut oil, and 1/2 tsp of cinnamon. Mix until the mixture resembles coarse crumbs.
5. Sprinkle the oat topping evenly over the apple filling.

Baking:

6. Bake the apple crisp for 30•35 minutes, or until the apples are tender and the topping is golden brown.
7. Allow the crisp to cool for 10•15 minutes before serving.

Serve the warm apple crisp on its own or with a scoop of vanilla ice cream or a dollop of whipped cream. The sweet, tender apples paired with the crunchy, nutty topping make for a delicious and comforting dessert.

86. Coconut Macaroons: Shredded coconut, egg whites, honey, vanilla extract, dark chocolate.

Ingredient:

- 2 cups unsweetened shredded coconut
- 2 egg whites
- 1/4 cup honey
- 1 tsp vanilla extract
- 1/4 cup dark chocolate chips or chopped dark chocolate

Instructions:

1. Preheat your oven to 325°F (165°C). Line a baking sheet with parchment paper.

2. In a medium bowl, whisk the egg whites until they are frothy.

3. Add the honey and vanilla extract to the egg whites and whisk until well combined.

4. Fold in the shredded coconut until it is evenly coated with the egg white mixture.

5. Scoop the coconut mixture by the tablespoonful and place them about 1 inch apart on the prepared baking sheet.

6. Bake for 15•18 minutes, or until the macaroons are lightly golden brown on the edges.

7. Remove the macaroons from the oven and let them cool on the baking sheet for 5 minutes.

8. Melt the dark chocolate in a double boiler or in the microwave, stirring frequently until smooth.

9. Drizzle the melted chocolate over the cooled macaroons.

10. Allow the chocolate to set before serving.

These Coconut Macaroons are chewy, sweet, and dipped in rich dark chocolate. The honey adds natural sweetness, while the vanilla enhances the coconut flavor.

Store the macaroons in an airtight container at room temperature for up to 1 week.

87. Peanut Butter Cookies:
Peanut butter, egg, honey, vanilla extract, baking soda.

Ingredient:

- 1 cup creamy peanut butter
- 1 egg
- 1/4 cup honey
- 1 tsp vanilla extract
- 1/2 tsp baking soda

Instructions:

1. Preheat your oven to 350°F (175°C). Line a baking sheet with parchment paper.

2. In a medium bowl, combine the peanut butter, egg, honey, vanilla extract, and baking soda. Mix until the ingredients are well incorporated and a smooth dough forms.

3. Scoop the dough by the tablespoonful and roll into balls. Place the balls about 2 inches apart on the prepared baking sheet.

4. Use a fork to gently press down on each cookie, creating a criss•cross pattern on the top.

5. Bake the cookies for 8•10 minutes, or until they are lightly golden around the edges.

6. Remove the cookies from the oven and let them cool on the baking sheet for 5 minutes before transferring them to a wire rack to cool completely.

These peanut butter cookies are soft, chewy, and naturally sweetened with honey. The baking soda helps them hold their shape and gives them a slightly crisp edge.

Store the cooled cookies in an airtight container at room temperature for up to 1 week.

Enjoy your homemade Peanut Butter Cookies!

88. Chocolate•Covered Strawberries:
Strawberries, dark chocolate, coconut oil, sea salt, honey.

Ingredient:

- 1 lb fresh strawberries, washed and patted dry
- 8 oz dark chocolate, chopped
- 1 tbsp coconut oil
- 1 tbsp honey
- 1/4 tsp sea salt

Instructions:

1. Line a baking sheet with parchment paper or a silicone baking mat.

2. In a double boiler or a heatproof bowl set over a saucepan of simmering water, melt the dark chocolate and coconut oil, stirring frequently until smooth.

3. Remove the chocolate mixture from the heat and stir in the honey until well combined.

4. Holding them by the stem, dip each strawberry into the melted chocolate, coating it completely.

5. Gently tap off any excess chocolate and place the chocolate•covered strawberries on the prepared baking sheet.

6. Sprinkle the sea salt over the top of the chocolate•covered strawberries.

7. Refrigerate the strawberries for at least 30 minutes, or until the chocolate has set.

The combination of sweet, juicy strawberries and rich, dark chocolate is simply irresistible. The coconut oil helps the chocolate set up nicely, while the honey adds a touch of sweetness. The sea salt provides a lovely contrast to the sweetness.

These Chocolate•Covered Strawberries make a beautiful and delicious treat for any occasion. Enjoy them chilled or at room temperature.

89. Baked Apples:
Apples, cinnamon, honey, almond flour, walnuts.

Ingredient:

- 4 medium•sized apples (such as Honeycrisp, Gala, or Fuji)
- 1/4 cup almond flour
- 2 tbsp honey
- 1 tsp ground cinnamon
- 1/4 cup chopped walnuts

Instructions:

1. Preheat your oven to 375°F (190°C).

2. Wash the apples and use a sharp knife or apple corer to cut off the top 1/4 of each apple and scoop out the core, leaving a well in the center.

3. In a small bowl, mix together the almond flour, honey, and cinnamon until well combined.

4. Spoon the almond flour mixture evenly into the hollowed•out centers of the apples.

5. Top each stuffed apple with a sprinkle of the chopped walnuts.

6. Place the stuffed apples in a baking dish and pour a small amount of water (about 1/4 cup) into the bottom of the dish.

7. Bake the apples for 30•35 minutes, or until they are tender when pierced with a fork.

8. Remove the baked apples from the oven and let them cool for 5•10 minutes before serving.

Serve the warm, baked apples on their own or with a dollop of whipped cream or a scoop of vanilla ice cream. The sweet, cinnamon•spiced filling pairs perfectly with the soft, baked apple.

Enjoy your homemade Baked Apples!

90. Berry Sorbet:
Mixed berries, honey, lemon juice, water, mint.

Ingredient:

- 3 cups mixed berries (such as strawberries, raspberries, blackberries)
- 1/4 cup honey
- 2 tbsp lemon juice
- 1/4 cup water
- 2 tbsp chopped fresh mint leaves

Instructions:

1. In a medium saucepan, combine the mixed berries, honey, lemon juice, and water. Bring the mixture to a simmer over medium heat, stirring occasionally, until the honey has dissolved and the berries have softened, about 5•7 minutes.

2. Remove the saucepan from the heat and let the berry mixture cool slightly.

3. Transfer the berry mixture to a blender or food processor and blend until smooth and pureed.

4. Pour the berry puree into a shallow baking dish or pan and place it in the freezer. Stir the mixture every 30 minutes for the first 2 hours to prevent large ice crystals from forming.

5. Once the sorbet has partially frozen, after about 2•3 hours, transfer it to a food processor or high•powered blender and blend until smooth and creamy.

6. Return the sorbet to the baking dish and continue freezing, stirring every 30 minutes, until it reaches your desired consistency, about 4•6 hours total.

7. Scoop the berry sorbet into serving bowls or cups and garnish with the chopped fresh mint leaves.

Serve the Berry Sorbet immediately or store it in an airtight container in the freezer for up to 2 weeks.

The combination of sweet berries, tart lemon, and refreshing mint creates a delightful and healthy frozen treat. Enjoy!

91. Protein Brownies: Protein powder, almond flour, cocoa powder, honey, eggs.

Ingredient:

- 1/2 cup almond flour
- 1/4 cup unsweetened cocoa powder
- 1/4 cup vanilla protein powder
- 1/4 tsp baking soda
- 1/4 tsp salt
- 2 eggs
- 1/4 cup honey
- 2 tbsp coconut oil, melted

Instructions:

1. Preheat your oven to 350°F (175°C). Grease an 8x8 inch baking pan.

2. In a medium bowl, whisk together the almond flour, cocoa powder, protein powder, baking soda, and salt.

3. In a separate bowl, beat the eggs. Then stir in the honey and melted coconut oil until well combined.

4. Pour the wet ingredients into the dry ingredients and mix until just combined, being careful not to overmix.

5. Spread the batter evenly into the prepared baking pan.

6. Bake for 18•22 minutes, or until a toothpick inserted in the center comes out clean.

7. Allow the brownies to cool completely in the pan before cutting into squares.

These Protein Brownies are fudgy, chocolatey, and packed with protein from the protein powder. The almond flour and honey provide a healthier alternative to traditional brownies.

You can use your choice of vanilla, chocolate, or even peanut butter protein powder to customize the flavor. Enjoy these guilt•free protein•packed treats!

92. Fruit Salad with Mint:
Mixed fruit, honey, lime juice, mint, chia seeds.

Ingredient:

- 2 cups mixed fruit (such as diced pineapple, mango, strawberries, blueberries, kiwi)
- 2 tbsp honey
- 1 tbsp fresh lime juice
- 2 tbsp chopped fresh mint leaves
- 1 tsp chia seeds

Instructions:

1. In a large bowl, gently toss together the mixed fruit.

2. In a small bowl, whisk together the honey and lime juice until well combined.

3. Drizzle the honey•lime dressing over the fruit and toss to coat evenly.

4. Sprinkle the chopped mint leaves and chia seeds over the top of the fruit salad.

5. Cover and refrigerate the fruit salad for at least 30 minutes to allow the flavors to meld.

6. Serve the chilled fruit salad as a refreshing side dish or healthy snack.

The combination of sweet, juicy fruit, tangy lime, and fragrant mint creates a delightful flavor profile. The chia seeds add a nutritional boost with their fiber, protein, and omega•3 content.

You can use any variety of fresh, seasonal fruits that you prefer. The honey•lime dressing complements a wide range of fruit combinations.

This Fruit Salad with Mint makes a great addition to brunch, picnics, or as a light dessert. Enjoy!

93. Oatmeal Cookies:
Oats, almond flour, honey, coconut oil, raisins.

Ingredient:

- 1 1/2 cups old•fashioned oats
- 1/2 cup almond flour
- 1/4 cup honey
- 1/4 cup coconut oil, melted
- 1 egg
- 1 tsp vanilla extract
- 1/2 tsp baking soda
- 1/4 tsp salt
- 1/2 cup raisins

Instructions:

1. Preheat your oven to 350°F (175°C). Line a baking sheet with parchment paper.

2. In a medium bowl, stir together the oats, almond flour, baking soda, and salt.

3. In a separate bowl, whisk together the honey, melted coconut oil, egg, and vanilla extract.

4. Pour the wet ingredients into the dry ingredients and mix until just combined. Fold in the raisins.

5. Scoop the dough by the tablespoonful and place the cookies about 2 inches apart on the prepared baking sheet.

6. Bake for 12•15 minutes, or until the cookies are lightly golden around the edges.

7. Allow the cookies to cool on the baking sheet for 5 minutes before transferring them to a wire rack to cool completely.

These Oatmeal Cookies are chewy, naturally sweetened, and packed with wholesome ingredients. The oats provide fiber, the almond flour adds protein, and the raisins offer a touch of sweetness.

Store the cooled cookies in an airtight container at room temperature for up to 1 week.

Enjoy your homemade Healthy Oatmeal Cookies!

94. Lemon Bars:
Almond flour, honey, eggs, lemon juice, coconut oil.

Ingredient:

- 1 1/2 cups almond flour
- 2 tbsp honey
- 2 tbsp coconut oil, melted

Filling Ingredients:
- 3 eggs
- 1/2 cup honey
- 1/2 cup fresh lemon juice (about 2•3 lemons)
- 2 tbsp almond flour
- 1 tbsp coconut oil, melted

Instructions:
For the Crust:
1. Preheat the oven to 350°F (175°C). Line an 8x8 inch baking pan with parchment paper.
2. In a medium bowl, mix together the almond flour, 2 tbsp honey, and 2 tbsp melted coconut oil until a dough forms.
3. Press the dough evenly into the bottom of the prepared baking pan.
4. Bake for 12•15 minutes, until lightly golden. Allow to cool.

For the Filling:

5. In a medium bowl, whisk together the eggs, 1/2 cup honey, lemon juice, 2 tbsp almond flour, and 1 tbsp melted coconut oil until well combined.
6. Pour the lemon filling over the cooled crust.
7. Bake for 18•22 minutes, until the center is set.
8. Allow the lemon bars to cool completely, then refrigerate for at least 2 hours before cutting into squares.

Serve chilled. Enjoy your healthier Lemon Bars!

The almond flour crust and honey•sweetened filling make these lemon bars a more nutritious treat. The coconut oil adds healthy fats, while the fresh lemon juice provides a bright, tangy flavor.

95. Mango Sorbet:
Mango, honey, lime juice, water, mint.

Ingredient:

- 3 cups diced fresh mango (about 2•3 mangoes)
- 1/4 cup honey
- 2 tbsp fresh lime juice
- 1/4 cup water
- 2 tbsp chopped fresh mint leaves

Instructions:

1. In a medium saucepan, combine the diced mango, honey, lime juice, and water. Bring the mixture to a simmer over medium heat, stirring occasionally, until the honey has dissolved, about 5 minutes.

2. Remove the saucepan from the heat and let the mango mixture cool slightly.

3. Transfer the mango mixture to a blender or food processor and blend until smooth and creamy.

4. Pour the mango puree into a shallow baking dish or pan and place it in the freezer. Stir the mixture every 30 minutes for the first 2 hours to prevent large ice crystals from forming.

5. Once the sorbet has partially frozen, after about 2•3 hours, transfer it to a food processor or high•powered blender and blend until smooth and creamy.

6. Return the sorbet to the baking dish and continue freezing, stirring every 30 minutes, until it reaches your desired consistency, about 4•6 hours total.

7. Scoop the mango sorbet into serving bowls or cups and garnish with the chopped fresh mint leaves.

Serve the Mango Sorbet immediately or store it in an airtight container in the freezer for up to 2 weeks.

The sweet, tropical flavor of the mango paired with the tart lime and refreshing mint creates a delightful and healthy frozen treat. Enjoy!

96. Pumpkin Pie Bites: Pumpkin puree, almond flour, honey, cinnamon, coconut oil.

Ingredient:

- 1 cup pumpkin puree
- 1 cup almond flour
- 1/4 cup honey
- 2 tbsp coconut oil, melted
- 1 tsp ground cinnamon
- 1/4 tsp ground nutmeg
- 1/4 tsp salt

Instructions:

1. In a medium bowl, combine the pumpkin puree, almond flour, honey, melted coconut oil, cinnamon, nutmeg, and salt. Mix until all the ingredients are well incorporated and a dough•like consistency forms.

2. Using a small cookie scoop or spoon, form the pumpkin mixture into bite•sized balls and place them on a parchment•lined baking sheet.

3. Refrigerate the pumpkin pie bites for at least 30 minutes to allow them to firm up.

4. Serve chilled or at room temperature.

These Pumpkin Pie Bites are a healthy, no•bake treat that captures the flavors of classic pumpkin pie. The pumpkin puree provides moisture and natural sweetness, while the almond flour, honey, and coconut oil bind the ingredients together.

The warm spices of cinnamon and nutmeg complement the pumpkin perfectly, creating a delicious and satisfying bite•sized dessert.

Store the pumpkin pie bites in an airtight container in the refrigerator for up to 1 week.

Enjoy your homemade Pumpkin Pie Bites!

97. Carrot Cake Bites: Carrots, almond flour, honey, cinnamon, coconut oil.

Ingredient:

- 1 cup grated carrots (about 2•3 medium carrots)
- 1 cup almond flour
- 1/4 cup honey
- 2 tbsp coconut oil, melted
- 1 tsp ground cinnamon
- 1/4 tsp salt

Instructions:

1. In a food processor, pulse the grated carrots until they are finely chopped and resemble a coarse texture.

2. In a medium bowl, combine the chopped carrots, almond flour, honey, melted coconut oil, cinnamon, and salt. Mix until all the ingredients are well incorporated and a dough•like consistency forms.

3. Using a small cookie scoop or spoon, form the mixture into bite•sized balls and place them on a parchment•lined baking sheet.

4. Refrigerate the carrot cake bites for at least 30 minutes to allow them to firm up.

5. Serve chilled or at room temperature.

These Carrot Cake Bites are a healthy, no•bake treat that satisfies your sweet tooth. The grated carrots provide moisture and natural sweetness, while the almond flour, honey, and coconut oil bind the ingredients together.

The cinnamon adds a warm, spiced flavor that complements the carrots perfectly. These bites make a great snack or dessert.

Store the carrot cake bites in an airtight container in the refrigerator for up to 1 week.

Enjoy your homemade Carrot Cake Bites!

98. Blueberry Muffins:
Almond flour, eggs, honey, blueberries, baking powder.

Ingredient:

- 2 cups almond flour
- 3 eggs
- 1/4 cup honey
- 1 tsp baking powder
- 1/4 tsp salt
- 1 cup fresh or frozen blueberries

Instructions:

1. Preheat your oven to 350°F (175°C). Grease a 12•cup muffin tin or line it with paper liners.

2. In a large bowl, whisk together the almond flour, baking powder, and salt.

3. In a separate bowl, beat the eggs and then stir in the honey.

4. Pour the wet ingredients into the dry ingredients and mix until just combined, being careful not to overmix.

5. Gently fold in the blueberries.

6. Scoop the batter evenly into the prepared muffin cups, filling them about 3/4 full.

7. Bake for 18•22 minutes, or until a toothpick inserted into the center comes out clean.

8. Allow the muffins to cool in the tin for 5 minutes before transferring them to a wire rack to cool completely.

These Blueberry Muffins are made with wholesome almond flour instead of traditional wheat flour, making them gluten•free and lower in carbs. The honey provides natural sweetness, and the blueberries add a burst of juicy flavor.

Store the cooled muffins in an airtight container at room temperature for up to 4 days, or in the freezer for up to 3 months.

Enjoy your homemade Healthy Blueberry Muffins!

99. Chocolate Peanut Butter Fudge: Peanut butter, cocoa powder, honey, coconut oil, vanilla extract.

Ingredient:

- 1 cup creamy peanut butter
- 1/2 cup unsweetened cocoa powder
- 1/4 cup honey
- 2 tbsp coconut oil, melted
- 1 tsp vanilla extract
- Pinch of salt

Instructions:

1. Line an 8x8 inch baking pan with parchment paper, leaving some overhang on the sides for easy removal.

2. In a medium bowl, whisk together the peanut butter, cocoa powder, honey, melted coconut oil, vanilla extract, and a pinch of salt until the mixture is smooth and well combined.

3. Spread the fudge mixture evenly into the prepared baking pan, smoothing the top with a spatula.

4. Refrigerate the fudge for at least 2 hours, or until it has completely set.

5. Once set, lift the fudge out of the pan using the parchment paper overhang. Peel off the paper and cut the fudge into small squares.

6. Store the chocolate peanut butter fudge in an airtight container in the refrigerator for up to 1 week.

This fudge is rich, creamy, and packed with the delicious combination of chocolate and peanut butter. The honey provides natural sweetness, while the coconut oil helps the fudge set up nicely.

Enjoy this healthier, homemade version of chocolate peanut butter fudge as a guilt•free treat or dessert.

100. Raspberry Chia Jam: Raspberries, chia seeds, honey, lemon juice, vanilla extract.

Ingredient:

- 2 cups fresh or frozen raspberries
- 2 tbsp chia seeds
- 2 tbsp honey
- 1 tbsp fresh lemon juice
- 1 tsp vanilla extract

Instructions:

1. In a medium saucepan, combine the raspberries, honey, lemon juice, and vanilla extract. Bring the mixture to a simmer over medium heat, stirring occasionally, until the raspberries have broken down, about 5•7 minutes.

2. Remove the saucepan from the heat and stir in the chia seeds. Make sure the chia seeds are evenly distributed throughout the raspberry mixture.

3. Transfer the raspberry chia jam to a clean jar or airtight container. Allow it to cool to room temperature, then refrigerate for at least 2 hours, or until the jam has thickened.

4. Once the jam has set, it's ready to use. Stir it before serving, as the chia seeds may cause the jam to separate slightly.

The raspberry chia jam can be used as a topping for toast, waffles, yogurt, or even as a filling for baked goods. It's a naturally sweetened, nutrient•dense alternative to store•bought jams.

Store the raspberry chia jam in the refrigerator for up to 1 week.

Enjoy your homemade Raspberry Chia Jam!

101. Green Juice:
Spinach, cucumber, apple, lemon, ginger.

Ingredient:

- 2 cups packed spinach leaves
- 1 medium cucumber, peeled and chopped
- 1 medium apple, cored and chopped
- 1 lemon, juiced
- 1•inch piece of fresh ginger, peeled and grated

Instructions:

1. Add the spinach, cucumber, apple, lemon juice, and grated ginger to a high•powered blender or juicer.

2. Blend or juice the ingredients until smooth and well combined.

3. If using a blender, you may need to add 1•2 tablespoons of water to help the mixture blend more easily.

4. Pour the green juice into a glass and enjoy immediately.

This green juice is packed with nutrients from the spinach, cucumber, apple, lemon, and ginger. The spinach provides vitamins, minerals, and antioxidants, the cucumber hydrates, the apple adds natural sweetness, the lemon provides a refreshing tartness, and the ginger adds a spicy kick.

You can adjust the amounts of each ingredient to suit your taste preferences. Some people also like to add a small handful of parsley or kale for an extra nutrient boost.

Drink the green juice immediately for maximum freshness and nutrient retention. Enjoy this healthy and refreshing beverage!

102. Berry Smoothie: Mixed berries, almond milk, honey, Greek yogurt, chia seeds.

Ingredient:

- 1 cup mixed berries (such as strawberries, blueberries, raspberries)
- 1 cup unsweetened almond milk
- 1/2 cup plain Greek yogurt
- 1 tbsp honey
- 1 tbsp chia seeds

Instructions:

1. Add all the ingredients to a high•powered blender.

2. Blend on high speed until the mixture is smooth and creamy, about 1•2 minutes.

3. Pour the berry smoothie into a glass and enjoy immediately.

This Berry Smoothie is a nutritious and delicious way to start your day or enjoy as a healthy snack. The mixed berries provide antioxidants, fiber, and natural sweetness. The almond milk adds creaminess and calcium, the Greek yogurt contributes protein, the honey sweetens it up, and the chia seeds offer omega•3s and fiber.

You can customize the smoothie by using different types of berries, adding a handful of spinach or kale for extra nutrients, or using vanilla or plain protein powder for an extra protein boost.

Enjoy your homemade Berry Smoothie!

103. Protein Shake: Protein powder, almond milk, banana, peanut butter, ice.

Ingredient:

- 1 scoop vanilla or chocolate protein powder
- 1 cup unsweetened almond milk
- 1 medium banana, frozen
- 2 tbsp creamy peanut butter
- 1 cup ice cubes

Instructions:

1. Add all the ingredients to a high•powered blender.

2. Blend on high speed until the mixture is smooth and creamy, about 1•2 minutes.

3. Pour the protein shake into a glass and enjoy immediately.

This Protein Shake is a great way to get a nutritious and filling snack or meal replacement. The protein powder provides a boost of protein to help build and repair muscle. The almond milk adds creaminess and calcium, the banana offers natural sweetness and potassium, the peanut butter contributes healthy fats and more protein, and the ice cubes help create a thick, milkshake•like texture.

You can customize the shake by using different types of protein powder, nut butters, or even adding a handful of spinach or kale for extra nutrients.

Enjoy your homemade Protein Shake!

104. Detox Water:
Water, cucumber, lemon, mint, ginger.

Ingredient:

- 1 cucumber, sliced
- 1 lemon, sliced
- 10•12 fresh mint leaves
- 1•inch piece of fresh ginger, peeled and sliced

Instructions:

1. In a large pitcher or water bottle, combine the sliced cucumber, lemon, mint leaves, and ginger slices.

2. Fill the pitcher or bottle with fresh, cold water.

3. Refrigerate the detox water for at least 2 hours, or up to 24 hours, to allow the flavors to infuse the water.

4. Serve the detox water chilled, making sure to include some of the cucumber, lemon, mint, and ginger slices in each glass.

5. Refill the pitcher or bottle with more water as needed, and continue to refrigerate for up to 3 days.

This Detox Water is a refreshing and healthy way to stay hydrated. The cucumber provides hydration and vitamins, the lemon adds a tart flavor and vitamin C, the mint leaves offer a refreshing aroma and flavor, and the ginger has anti•inflammatory properties.

Drinking this infused water throughout the day can help flush out toxins, aid digestion, and provide a boost of antioxidants. You can also experiment with other fruit and herb combinations, such as strawberry and basil or orange and rosemary.

Enjoy your homemade Detox Water!

105. Iced Coffee:
Coffee, almond milk, honey, vanilla extract, ice.

Ingredient:

- 1 cup brewed coffee, cooled
- 1 cup unsweetened almond milk
- 1•2 tbsp honey (or to taste)
- 1 tsp vanilla extract
- Ice cubes

Instructions:

1. In a pitcher or large glass, combine the cooled coffee, almond milk, honey, and vanilla extract. Stir until the honey is fully dissolved.

2. Fill a glass with ice cubes.

3. Pour the iced coffee mixture over the ice.

4. Stir gently and enjoy immediately.

You can adjust the amounts of almond milk and honey to suit your taste preferences. Start with 1 tbsp of honey and add more if you'd like it sweeter.

The almond milk provides a creamy, dairy•free base, while the honey adds natural sweetness. The vanilla extract enhances the flavor of the coffee.

This Iced Coffee is a refreshing and healthier alternative to traditional iced coffee drinks. It's perfect for a hot day or as an afternoon pick•me•up.

You can also make a larger batch and store it in the refrigerator for up to 5 days, giving you easy access to a delicious iced coffee whenever you need it.

Enjoy your homemade Iced Coffee!

106. Mango Smoothie:
Mango, almond milk, honey, Greek yogurt, ice.

Ingredient:

- 1 cup frozen mango chunks
- 1 cup unsweetened almond milk
- 1/2 cup plain Greek yogurt
- 1 tbsp honey (or to taste)
- 1 cup ice cubes

Instructions:

1. Add all the ingredients to a high•powered blender.

2. Blend on high speed until the mixture is smooth and creamy, about 1•2 minutes.

3. Pour the mango smoothie into a glass and enjoy immediately.

This Mango Smoothie is a delicious and nutritious way to start your day or enjoy as a healthy snack. The frozen mango provides natural sweetness, fiber, and vitamins. The almond milk adds creaminess and calcium, the Greek yogurt contributes protein, and the honey sweetens it up.

You can customize the smoothie by using different types of yogurt, adding a handful of spinach or kale for extra nutrients, or using vanilla or plain protein powder for an extra protein boost.

Enjoy your homemade Mango Smoothie!

107. Hot Chocolate: Almond milk, cocoa powder, honey, vanilla extract, cinnamon.

Ingredient:

- 2 cups unsweetened almond milk
- 2 tbsp unsweetened cocoa powder
- 1•2 tbsp honey (to taste)
- 1 tsp vanilla extract
- 1/4 tsp ground cinnamon

Instructions:

1. In a small saucepan, whisk together the almond milk, cocoa powder, honey, vanilla extract, and cinnamon.

2. Heat the mixture over medium heat, whisking frequently, until it's hot and well combined, about 5 minutes. Do not boil.

3. Remove the saucepan from the heat.

4. Pour the hot chocolate into mugs.

5. Optionally, you can top the hot chocolate with a sprinkle of additional cinnamon or a dollop of whipped cream.

This Healthy Hot Chocolate is a delicious and comforting treat that's made with wholesome ingredients. The almond milk provides a creamy base, the cocoa powder gives it a rich chocolate flavor, the honey sweetens it naturally, the vanilla enhances the flavor, and the cinnamon adds a warm, spiced note.

You can adjust the amount of honey to your desired sweetness level. This recipe is dairy•free, but you can also use regular milk if preferred.

Enjoy your homemade Healthy Hot Chocolate!

108. Pineapple Smoothie:
Pineapple, coconut milk, honey, Greek yogurt, ice.

Ingredient:

- 1 cup fresh or frozen pineapple chunks
- 1 cup milk (dairy, almond, or oat milk)
- 1/2 cup plain Greek yogurt
- 1 tbsp honey (optional)
- 1/2 tsp vanilla extract
- 1 cup ice cubes

Instructions:

1. Add all the ingredients to a blender • the pineapple, milk, yogurt, honey (if using), vanilla, and ice cubes.

2. Blend on high speed until smooth and creamy, about 1•2 minutes.

3. Pour into a glass and enjoy immediately.

Optional Variations:

- Add a banana for extra creaminess
- Use coconut milk instead of regular milk
- Blend in a handful of spinach or kale for extra nutrients
- Top with shredded coconut, granola, or a pineapple wedge

This pineapple smoothie is refreshing, packed with vitamins and protein, and makes a great breakfast or snack. Adjust the ingredients to your taste preferences. Enjoy!

109. Herbal Tea:
Herbal tea bag, hot water, honey, lemon, mint.

Ingredient:

- 1 herbal tea bag (such as chamomile, peppermint, or ginger)
- 1 cup hot water
- 1•2 tsp honey (to taste)
- 1 slice of lemon
- 2•3 fresh mint leaves (optional)

Instructions:

1. Bring 1 cup of water to a boil.

2. Place the herbal tea bag in a mug or teapot. Pour the hot water over the tea bag.

3. Let the tea steep for 5•7 minutes, allowing the flavors to infuse the water.

4. Remove the tea bag and stir in 1•2 teaspoons of honey, to taste. The honey will help sweeten and soothe the tea.

5. Add a slice of lemon and 2•3 fresh mint leaves (if using). The lemon and mint provide a refreshing, aromatic element.

6. Enjoy the herbal tea hot. You can add more honey or lemon to adjust the flavor to your liking.

Some herbal tea options to try:

- Chamomile • calming and soothing
- Peppermint • refreshing and aids digestion
- Ginger • warming and can help with nausea
- Hibiscus • tart and high in vitamin C

Herbal teas are a great way to relax, stay hydrated, and support overall wellness. Customize this recipe with your favorite herbal tea blend.

110. Apple Cider:
Apple juice, cinnamon sticks, cloves, nutmeg, honey.

Ingredient:

- 4 cups apple juice or cider
- 2 cinnamon sticks
- 4•5 whole cloves
- 1/4 tsp ground nutmeg
- 1•2 tbsp honey (to taste)

Instructions:

1. In a medium saucepan, combine the apple juice/cider, cinnamon sticks, cloves, and nutmeg.

2. Bring the mixture to a simmer over medium heat. Once simmering, reduce the heat to low and let it steep for 15•20 minutes, allowing the flavors to infuse.

3. Remove the saucepan from the heat and stir in 1•2 tablespoons of honey, to taste. The honey will help sweeten and balance the flavors.

4. Strain the cider through a fine mesh sieve to remove the cinnamon sticks and cloves.

5. Serve the apple cider warm, either in mugs or heat•safe glasses. You can garnish with an extra cinnamon stick or a slice of apple, if desired.

Optional Variations:

- Use a combination of apple juice and apple cider for a more robust flavor.
- Add a few slices of fresh ginger for a spicy kick.
- Stir in a splash of brandy or rum for an adult version.
- Top with a dollop of whipped cream or a sprinkle of ground cinnamon.

This homemade apple cider is perfect for chilly autumn and winter days. The blend of spices and honey creates a cozy, comforting beverage. Enjoy!

111. Protein Coffee:
Coffee, protein powder, almond milk, honey, ice.

Ingredient:

- 1 cup brewed coffee, cooled
- 1•2 scoops protein powder (vanilla or chocolate flavor)
- 1/2 cup unsweetened almond milk
- 1•2 tsp honey (to taste)
- Ice cubes

Instructions:

1. In a blender, combine the brewed coffee, protein powder, almond milk, and honey.

2. Blend on high speed until the mixture is smooth and frothy, about 30 seconds to 1 minute.

3. Add ice cubes to a glass.

4. Pour the protein coffee over the ice.

5. Stir gently to combine.

6. Enjoy the protein coffee immediately.

Optional Variations:

- Use a different type of milk, such as regular milk, oat milk, or coconut milk.
- Add a banana or a spoonful of peanut butter for extra creaminess and nutrients.
- Sprinkle a dash of cinnamon or cocoa powder on top.
- Swap the honey for maple syrup or agave nectar.

This protein coffee is a great way to start your day with a boost of energy and protein. The combination of coffee, protein powder, and almond milk creates a creamy, satisfying drink. Adjust the sweetener and protein powder amount to your personal taste preferences.

112. Coconut Water:
Coconut water, lime juice, mint, honey, ice.

Ingredient:

- 1 cup coconut water
- 2 tbsp fresh lime juice
- 1•2 tsp honey (to taste)
- 4•5 fresh mint leaves
- Ice cubes

Instructions:

1. In a glass, combine the coconut water, lime juice, and honey. Stir well until the honey is fully dissolved.

2. Gently bruise the mint leaves with the back of a spoon to release the oils and aroma. Add the mint leaves to the glass.

3. Fill the glass with ice cubes.

4. Stir the mixture again to combine all the Ingredients.

5. Garnish with an extra mint sprig, if desired.

6. Serve immediately and enjoy!

Optional Variations:

- Add a splash of club soda or sparkling water for some fizz.
- Use a combination of coconut water and pineapple juice.
- Muddle a few slices of cucumber in the glass before adding the other ingredients.
- Rim the glass with a lime wedge and dip in shredded coconut.

This coconut water mocktail is a refreshing, hydrating, and lightly sweetened beverage. The lime juice and mint provide a bright, tropical flavor profile. Adjust the honey to your desired sweetness level. Enjoy this healthy and delicious drink!

113. Avocado Smoothie:
Avocado, almond milk, honey, Greek yogurt, ice.

Ingredient:

- 1 ripe avocado, pitted and peeled
- 1 cup unsweetened almond milk
- 1/2 cup plain Greek yogurt
- 1•2 tbsp honey (to taste)
- 1 cup ice cubes

Instructions:

1. In a blender, combine the avocado, almond milk, Greek yogurt, and honey.

2. Blend on high speed until the mixture is smooth and creamy, about 1•2 minutes.

3. Add the ice cubes and blend again until the smoothie is thick and well•combined.

4. Taste and adjust sweetness by adding more honey if desired.

5. Pour the avocado smoothie into a glass and serve immediately.

Optional Variations:

- Use regular milk or another non•dairy milk instead of almond milk.
- Add a banana for extra creaminess and natural sweetness.
- Blend in a handful of spinach or kale for extra nutrients.
- Top with sliced avocado, toasted coconut, or a drizzle of honey.

This avocado smoothie is packed with healthy fats, protein, and vitamins. The avocado provides a rich, creamy texture, while the Greek yogurt and honey add a touch of sweetness. It makes a nutritious breakfast, snack, or post•workout recovery drink. Enjoy this delicious and nourishing smoothie!

114. Turmeric Latte: Almond milk, turmeric, honey, cinnamon, black pepper.

Ingredient:

- 1 cup unsweetened almond milk
- 1 tsp ground turmeric
- 1•2 tsp honey (to taste)
- 1/4 tsp ground cinnamon
- Pinch of ground black pepper

Instructions:

1. In a small saucepan, whisk together the almond milk, turmeric, honey, cinnamon, and black pepper.

2. Heat the mixture over medium heat, whisking frequently, until it is steaming hot but not boiling, about 2•3 minutes.

3. Remove the saucepan from the heat.

4. Using a milk frother or whisk, froth the heated milk mixture until it is foamy and frothy.

5. Pour the turmeric latte into a mug.

6. Optionally, you can top it with an extra sprinkle of cinnamon or a drizzle of honey.

7. Enjoy the warm, comforting turmeric latte immediately.

Optional Variations:

- Use regular dairy milk or another non•dairy milk like coconut or oat milk.
- Add a small pinch of ground ginger for extra warmth.
- Stir in a shot of espresso for a turmeric•spiced latte.
- Top with a sprinkle of nutmeg or cardamom.

The combination of turmeric, cinnamon, and black pepper creates a flavorful and anti•inflammatory latte. The honey adds a touch of sweetness to balance the earthy turmeric. Enjoy this cozy and nourishing drink any time of day.

115. Strawberry Smoothie:
Strawberries, almond milk, honey, Greek yogurt, ice.

Ingredient:

- 1 cup fresh or frozen strawberries
- 1 cup unsweetened almond milk
- 1/2 cup plain Greek yogurt
- 1•2 tbsp honey (to taste)
- 1 cup ice cubes

Instructions:

1. In a blender, combine the strawberries, almond milk, Greek yogurt, and honey.

2. Blend on high speed until the mixture is smooth and creamy, about 1•2 minutes.

3. Add the ice cubes and blend again until the smoothie is thick and well•combined.

4. Taste and adjust sweetness by adding more honey if desired.

5. Pour the strawberry smoothie into a glass and serve immediately.

Optional Variations:

- Use regular milk or another non•dairy milk instead of almond milk.
- Add a banana for extra creaminess and natural sweetness.
- Blend in a handful of spinach or kale for extra nutrients.
- Top with fresh strawberry slices, granola, or a drizzle of honey.

This strawberry smoothie is a refreshing and nutritious treat. The combination of sweet strawberries, creamy Greek yogurt, and almond milk creates a delightful flavor and texture. The honey adds a touch of sweetness to balance the tartness of the berries. Enjoy this smoothie as a healthy breakfast, snack, or post•workout recovery drink.

116. Matcha Latte: Matcha powder, almond milk, honey, vanilla extract, ice.

Ingredient:

- 1 tsp matcha green tea powder
- 1 cup unsweetened almond milk
- 1•2 tsp honey (to taste)
- 1/2 tsp vanilla extract
- Ice cubes (optional)

Instructions:

1. In a small bowl or mug, whisk the matcha powder with 2•3 tablespoons of the almond milk until it forms a smooth paste, without any lumps.

2. In a small saucepan, heat the remaining almond milk over medium heat, stirring frequently, until it is steaming hot but not boiling.

3. Remove the saucepan from the heat and pour the hot almond milk into the bowl with the matcha paste. Whisk vigorously until the mixture is frothy and well•combined.

4. Stir in the honey and vanilla extract, adjusting the sweetness to your taste.

5. If desired, pour the matcha latte over ice in a glass.

6. Enjoy the matcha latte immediately while it's hot and frothy.

Optional Variations:

- Use regular dairy milk or another non•dairy milk like oat or coconut milk.
- Add a sprinkle of cinnamon or nutmeg on top.
- Blend the latte in a high•speed blender for an extra frothy texture.
- Substitute the honey with maple syrup or agave nectar.

The combination of earthy matcha, creamy almond milk, and sweet honey creates a delightful and soothing latte. Matcha is packed with antioxidants and provides a gentle caffeine boost. Enjoy this healthy and comforting drink any time of day.

117. Lemon Ginger Tea:
Hot water, lemon, ginger, honey, mint.

Ingredient:

- 1 cup hot water
- 1 inch fresh ginger, peeled and sliced
- 1 lemon, juiced
- 1•2 tsp honey (to taste)
- 2•3 fresh mint leaves

Instructions:

1. In a mug or teapot, pour the hot water over the sliced ginger.

2. Let the ginger steep for 5•7 minutes to infuse the water with its flavor.

3. Remove the ginger slices and stir in the fresh lemon juice.

4. Add 1•2 teaspoons of honey, to taste, and stir until the honey is fully dissolved.

5. Gently bruise the mint leaves with the back of a spoon to release the oils, then add them to the tea.

6. Enjoy the lemon ginger tea hot, with the mint leaves providing a refreshing aroma.

Optional Variations:

- Use a combination of lemon and lime juice.
- Add a cinnamon stick or a few cloves for extra warmth.
- Steep a lemon or ginger tea bag instead of using fresh ingredients.
- Garnish with a lemon slice or extra mint leaves.

This lemon ginger tea is a soothing and nourishing beverage. The ginger provides a warming, slightly spicy flavor, while the lemon adds a bright, tangy note. The honey helps to balance the flavors and soothe the throat. Enjoy this comforting tea any time you need a pick•me•up or a moment of relaxation.

118. Peach Smoothie:
Peaches, almond milk, honey, Greek yogurt, ice.

Ingredient:

- 1 cup fresh or frozen peach slices
- 1 cup unsweetened almond milk
- 1/2 cup plain Greek yogurt
- 1•2 tbsp honey (to taste)
- 1 cup ice cubes

Instructions:

1. In a blender, combine the peach slices, almond milk, Greek yogurt, and honey.

2. Blend on high speed until the mixture is smooth and creamy, about 1•2 minutes.

3. Add the ice cubes and blend again until the smoothie is thick and well•combined.

4. Taste and adjust sweetness by adding more honey if desired.

5. Pour the peach smoothie into a glass and serve immediately.

Optional Variations:

- Use regular milk or another non•dairy milk instead of almond milk.
- Add a banana for extra creaminess and natural sweetness.
- Blend in a handful of spinach or kale for extra nutrients.
- Top with sliced fresh peaches, toasted almonds, or a drizzle of honey.

This peach smoothie is a refreshing and nutritious treat. The combination of sweet peaches, creamy Greek yogurt, and almond milk creates a delightful flavor and texture. The honey adds a touch of sweetness to balance the tartness of the peaches. Enjoy this smoothie as a healthy breakfast, snack, or post•workout recovery drink.

119. Beet Juice:
Beets, apple, lemon, ginger, water.

Ingredient:

- 2 medium•sized beets, peeled and chopped
- 1 apple, cored and chopped
- 1 inch fresh ginger, peeled
- 1 lemon, juiced
- 1/2 cup water (optional)

Instructions:

1. In a juicer, juice the beets, apple, and ginger. Alternatively, you can use a high•powered blender and then strain the mixture through a fine mesh sieve.

2. Stir in the freshly squeezed lemon juice.

3. If the juice is too thick, add up to 1/2 cup of water and stir to thin it out to your desired consistency.

4. Pour the beet juice into a glass and enjoy immediately.

Optional Variations:

- Add a handful of spinach or kale for extra nutrients.
- Substitute the apple with a carrot or orange for a different flavor profile.
- Stir in a teaspoon of honey or maple syrup for a touch of sweetness.
- Garnish with a slice of lemon or a sprig of fresh mint.

This beet juice is packed with vitamins, minerals, and antioxidants. The combination of sweet beets, tart lemon, and spicy ginger creates a vibrant and flavorful juice. Beets are known for their anti•inflammatory properties and ability to support detoxification. Enjoy this refreshing and healthy beet juice as part of a balanced diet.

As we reach the end of the **"5 Ingredient Cookbook for Men: Cooking Hacks for Men Who Hate Complicated Recipes,"** we hope you've discovered a newfound confidence and enjoyment in the kitchen. Cooking doesn't have to be daunting or time-consuming—it can be a rewarding experience that brings joy to you and those you cook for.

Throughout this journey, we've explored simple yet delicious recipes that prove you don't need a long list of ingredients to create impressive meals. Whether you've mastered the art of grilling a perfect steak with just a few seasonings or whipped up a decadent dessert in minutes, each dish has been crafted with your busy lifestyle in mind.

Remember, cooking is a skill that grows with practice. Embrace the creativity that comes with experimenting in the kitchen, and don't be afraid to put your own spin on our recipes. The key ingredients—simplicity, flavor, and enjoyment—are always at your disposal.

Thank you for choosing this cookbook as your guide. We hope it continues to inspire you to cook with passion, savor every bite, and share the joy of good food with those around you. Here's to many more delicious adventures in the kitchen!

Happy cooking